I AM WHOLE AGAIN

I AM WHOLE AGAIN

The Case for Breast Reconstruction after Mastectomy

Jean Zalon
with Jean Libman Block

Random House
New York

Copyright © 1978 by Jean Zalon and Jean Libman Block
All rights reserved under International and Pan-American Copyright Conventions.
Published in the United States by Random House, Inc., New York, and simultaneously in Canada by Random House of Canada Limited, Toronto.
Grateful acknowledgment is made to the following for permission to reprint previously published material:
The New York Times: Text as submitted by Dee Wedemeyer, December 9, 1976. © 1976 by The New York Times Company.

Library of Congress Cataloging in Publication Data

Zalon, Jean.
I am whole again.

1. Mammoplasty—Biography. 2. Zalon, Jean. 3. Mastectomy—Psychological aspects. I. Block, Jean Libman, joint author. II. Title.
RD539.8.Z34 618.1'9 77–90305
ISBN 0-394-42532-4

Manufactured in the United States of America
2 4 6 8 9 7 5 3
First Edition

Preface

Although only one woman in thirteen develops breast cancer, most women at some time will suffer from lumps, pain or nipple discharge sufficient to cause concern and warrant medical care. The fear of cancer is therefore widespread. Because the most commonly used treatment is mastectomy, the fear of the diagnosis of cancer is compounded by the fear of the treatment itself. In our breast-oriented society many women, particularly those under fifty, are often as much concerned about the loss of the breast as about the possible loss of life. One of the saddest experiences of the physician involved in women's breast care is the statement, "I'd rather take my chances with dying from breast cancer than have to suffer the emotional upheaval of losing a breast."

Jean Zalon, in her understanding, sympathetic approach to the woman faced with the possible loss of a breast, is emphasizing the potential answer to a highly emotional problem. Reconstruction after mastectomy—with proper guidelines in the selection of candidates—offers an acceptable solution to the terrible dilemma faced by a woman about to undergo breast surgery.

Assurance that a mastectomy can be performed in a manner that would permit a reconstruction in a reasonable length of time and "make a woman whole again" can bring considerable peace of mind. Add to such assurance an actual demonstration of a woman who has had a successful reconstruction, and a tremendous emotional load can be lifted from an extraordinarily distraught patient. This approach can prevent delay in treatment as well as "shopping around" in a potentially disastrous search for the physician who will agree to less than mastectomy.

It is time for the experience of an intelligent woman, who was fortunate enough to gain the knowledge of the procedure and to profit from the skill of an experienced plastic surgeon, to be made available to the general public. Women should read this book because it might be helpful to themselves as well as to others close to them.

Finally, it should be emphasized that the best results in the reconstruction are dependent on the stage of the disease when treated. The earlier the detection and the smaller the cancer, the greater the chance that the successful reconstruction will be possible. The concept of reconstruction emphasizes the need for more widespread knowledge that early detection of breast cancer can save lives. Now we can add: Early detection not only saves lives but makes it possible for a woman to be whole again.

—Philip Strax, M.D. (medical director, Guttman Breast Diagnostic Institute; director, Department of Radiology, La Guardia Hospital; associate clinical professor, Community and Preventive Medicine, New York Medical College)

Contents

		Preface by Philip Strax, M.D.	v
		Introduction	3
1	/	My Mastectomy	7
2	/	My Search for Reconstruction	23
3	/	The Start of My Reconstruction	29
4	/	My Reconstruction	42
5	/	Now, What about the Other Breast?	55
6	/	Whole, at Last	64
7	/	Going Public	70
8	/	Women Respond	83
9	/	The History of Reconstruction	93
10	/	The State of the Controversy	101
11	/	The Current State of the Art: Routine Procedures	107
12	/	The Current State of the Art: Complex Procedures	113
13	/	The Psychology of Breast Loss	120
14	/	What Can Be Done— on the Psychological Level	128
15	/	Time for Reconstruction	135
16	/	Questions Most Frequently Asked about Breast Reconstruction	143

I AM
WHOLE
AGAIN

Introduction

My search for the replacement of my left breast began soon after my mastectomy in 1970. Without the breast, I hated the way I looked. I felt both physically and psychologically spoiled and was unable to shake off a feeling of incompleteness and emptiness. There was a void in myself. In addition, the absence of the breast served as a constant reminder of the cancer that had once invaded my body and left me with a sense of dread and foreboding.

Why couldn't some facsimile of a breast be built on my body to restore the lost contours? I knew that plastic surgeons were routinely inserting little silicone pads under the breast tissue to enlarge the bosoms of women who felt that what nature had given them was inadequate. I also knew that overly large or excessively pendulous breasts could be reduced in size. I'd met a delightful young woman who'd had her flat, tiny breasts enhanced to shapely curves. "What's really great," she'd said with a mischievous smile, "is that I don't have to wear a sign any more that says, 'Front.'" I'd joined in the laughter that followed her remark, but my laugh was hollow and I cried that night.

I had even read somewhere that a transsexual wishing to change from male to female could have quite passable breasts created by plastic surgeons. And I'd heard of the reconstruction of the genitals of Russian soldiers wounded during World War II.

The surgical skills and techniques for making a breast seemed to be available. Why, then, couldn't I have my lost breast rebuilt?

It took nearly four disheartening and frustrating years before my dream could be fulfilled. When my new breast was finally built in 1974, I discovered that I had taken only a first step in a journey that was more complicated than I had imagined at the outset.

There was the question of reshaping my healthy right breast to match the reconstructed one on the left side. There was also the question of constructing a nipple for the new left breast. All these problems were resolved as they came along and I underwent the required operations in almost total loneliness. Nobody I knew had had breast reconstruction. I could find no books or magazine articles which described the experiences of women who had tried reconstruction or which discussed the advantages or disadvantages of such surgery.

My family was terrified that I was taking needless chances with my body and my life. My husband thought I was out of my mind for longing so desperately to replace the lost breast. My friends feared the risk of stirring up latent cancer cells. No counseling services were available to help me work out my emotional conflicts.

Worst of all, no one was around to tell me that it was *normal* to feel deprived after a breast amputation and *normal* to long for wholeness.

I took this lonely journey by myself. When I finally reached my goal, I was overwhelmed with happiness. My joy at the recaptured wholeness of my body was so great that it overflowed and I found myself reaching out to other women to tell them that for a great many of them deformity and the suffering caused by it were not necessary. A mastectomy need not be permanently maiming; the hiding of a woman's scarred body from herself and from others need not be a lifelong sentence to misery; a shattered self-image need not destroy the joys of sex and the warmth of close relationships.

The more I talked to women who had lost a breast and heard their stories of discontent and depression, the more urgently I wanted to spread the word of reconstruction. I went to medical libraries to arm myself with more information. I entered into correspondence with cancer surgeons and with plastic surgeons in various parts of the country to find out what techniques of reconstruction were being used and what results were being obtained. I interviewed social workers and psychiatrists to learn more about the emotional impact of breast loss on a woman and her family.

When the story of my own reconstruction was told in a major newspaper, the floodgates opened. Hundreds of women wrote me, called me, came to see me. They listened, astonished, to my story of reconstruction. They looked with wonder at what the plastic surgeon had accomplished for me. By this time my tears for myself had stopped, but I cried all over again with many of my visitors.

A large percentage of these women who had lost a breast had never heard of reconstruction. Some who had heard of it were fearful. Some had altogether erroneous ideas. Most were ashamed of their unhappiness over their disfigured bodies and were torn apart by the conflict between their unquenchable grief and the demands made by the world around them that they face their loss bravely.

I knew that beyond these women who found my address and telephone number there were many thousands of others who were searching for wholeness and for a way to come to terms with their altered bodies. The number of breast cancers diagnosed each year has reached 91,000; the number of women now alive who have lost a breast to cancer exceeds 500,000. All these women and the additional thousands who will hear the grim diagnosis in future months and years deserve to have the facts about reconstruction immediately available to them. Only with such knowledge can they make sensible and informed decisions about the steps to take next.

For breast reconstruction after mastectomy is an idea whose time is right now. Breast surgeons are now beginning to shed their reluctance to recommend reconstruction. Plastic surgeons are perfecting older techniques and developing newer ones. Social workers and psychologists are helping patients to sort out their tangled feelings over breast loss and replacement.

No one seems to have any exact figures about the number of reconstructions performed a year, but several expert estimates put the total well above 5,000 at this time, with a predicted annual doubling and tripling in the years immediately ahead.

I hope that my efforts on behalf of reconstruction have played at least a small part in the change to a more favorable attitude. And I hope also that this book will help persuade doctors, patients and their families that the case for breast reconstruction after mastectomy is strong and, indeed, compelling.

Of the dozens and dozens of women I've talked to in recent months, quite a few were willing to discuss in great detail their experiences and feelings related to the loss and rebuilding of their breasts. Some were willing for me to tape their frank revelations about the impact of their surgery on their marriages, their sex lives, their sense of self-worth.

From these tapes I have selected seven that represent a wide spectrum of attitudes and feelings. I have changed names and altered details to prevent embarrassment to the women and their families. But the events and the emotions are all true.

You will find records of these conversations throughout the book.

1

My Mastectomy

My story began in June 1970 in the shower. While I was washing myself I felt a small lump in the lower central part of my left breast below the nipple. I froze with absolute horror. Breast cancer was terribly familiar to me because I worked with it every day.

For the past ten years I had been employed at the Health Insurance Plan of New York, a prepaid medical service, that was carrying on a large-scale study to determine the value of x-ray screening, or mammography, in the early detection of breast cancer. Under a grant from the U.S. Public Health Service, HIP was conducting annual breast screenings of thirty thousand women. My job was to follow up cancer patients by means of hospital and doctors' records and through personal interviews.

The minute I was out of the shower I ran to the telephone and made an appointment to see Dr. Louis Venet the next day. Dr. Venet was the consultant on our breast cancer study; I knew and admired him. He was kind, thorough and most conscientious. I never hesitated for a moment on the choice of a doctor.

Naturally, I was upset and frightened. But I didn't panic the way some women do, because I knew from my work that the majority of breast tumors are benign.

"I don't think it's anything serious," Dr. Venet told me the next day, "but I'm not God and so there's no point in speculating. We'll have to take a biopsy." A biopsy is the removal of a small piece of the suspect tissue and its examination under powerful microscopes for evidence of malignant cells. If the problem is a cyst on or near the surface of the skin, an aspiration, or withdrawal of fluid, can be handled in the doctor's office. But if the trouble is a lump which lies inside the breast, then the procedure is done under full anesthesia in the hospital.

Mine would have to be done in the hospital.

I took the subway back to my office, and by this time I could feel the fear collecting inside me. But side by side with the fear was disbelief that anything really bad could happen to me. "I'm still invulnerable," I told myself. "It won't be anything."

My thoughts tried to be brave, but the terror was beginning to set in.

I told Bea, my closest friend at the office, that I had to have a lump biopsied. I expected sympathy from her, but she delivered it in such copious quantities and became so overwrought that one of the other women in the department urged her to take something to calm herself down. Bea took a sedative, and almost immediately she had a violent reaction to the medication, so violent that she became sick and fainted. One of the women in our department ran to find a doctor who was free. Another helped me drag Bea's limp body to his office. Three of us steadied her when, a few minutes later, her eyes fluttered open and she made her first tentative effort to sit and then to stand.

Once I was sure that Bea had recovered, I got mad. "Hey, you stole my scene," I told her indignantly. "That should have been my thing. If anyone's supposed to faint around here, I'm the one."

We all laughed and, at least momentarily, I was diverted from my problem.

I managed to stay reasonably calm in the office, but at home that night I let all my fear and anger spill out. My husband, Jules, a man of monumental calm, had to take wave after wave of my fury and terror. I'll spare you the details of my outburst —let your imagination fill them in.

The next day I went to see another doctor who was also connected with our breast cancer study. His opinion was the same as Dr. Venet's—I needed an immediate biopsy to find out about that little lump.

My admission to the hospital was not exactly uneventful. It is standard procedure for the patient who is to have a biopsy to sign a paper giving the surgeon permission to proceed with further surgery if necessary. Further surgery, of course, is mastectomy if the biopsy shows presence of cancer. What this means, then, is that the patient remains under anesthesia while the excised bit of tissue is rushed to the pathologist. He freezes the tissue, examines it under a microscope and telephones his findings to the waiting surgeon. If a malignancy is detected, the surgeon amputates the breast of the still-anesthetized patient.

I refused to sign that little piece of paper.

Looking back now, I sometimes wonder how I had the courage to defy tradition, hospital rules and my own surgeon's wishes. But I was adamant—no release for additional surgery. I had several reasons for my refusal. First, I didn't feel altogether secure about the accuracy of biopsy. In the course of my work I had learned that biopsy is really a two-stage procedure. First, there is the examination of the frozen section, usually done while the patient is still anesthetized. Later the suspect tissue is encased in paraffin and examined for a more detailed diagnosis of the type of cancer that is present. The paraffin study is usually made by the pathologist after the patient's surgery has been completed.

I had heard of a few isolated cases of biopsies that were misread or of instances when the later paraffin study contradicted the earlier frozen section. I knew that it was theoretically possible that a lesion could be pronounced benign rather than malignant—*after* the breast was amputated. I knew this possibility was unlikely, but even so, it made my blood run cold.

(Now we know that it is not all that unlikely, for only recently the National Cancer Institute has revealed that during its nationwide breast-screening project conducted over a four-year period, three women did have their breasts wholly or partly removed because of erroneous diagnosis of cancer. And an expert panel has now recommended that three pathologists should evaluate all suspected tumors before surgery is performed.)

However slight the chances of an unnecessary mastectomy appeared at that time, I still had enough doubt to want both types of biopsies read and even a confirming opinion of the findings by another pathologist before any irrevocable steps were taken.

My other reason for refusing to sign the permission slip was quite different and, in its way, even more important to me. I was determined to remain aware of and in control of whatever happened to me and my breast. I didn't want to come out of anesthesia and face a shocking, irreversible condition.

I wanted to go into anesthesia the first time knowing that the worst that could happen would be a verdict of cancer. I could not face the uncertainty of waking up, afraid to raise my hand to my breast for fear of what I would discover. If a mastectomy was really necessary, I wanted to make a conscious decision to have it done when I was in full possession of my faculties. To repeat, I could not tolerate going into the operating room just for a biopsy and finding out hours later that I no longer had a breast.

Dr. Venet had known of my intended refusal to sign the permission and had tried earlier to argue me out of my stubbornness. He'd pointed out that it would not be good for me to have anesthesia twice in the same week. I didn't care—I stood firm. Now, at the time I was to be admitted, hospital officials were giving me a hard time, insisting that no one before had taken this foolish stand. No matter what they said, I wouldn't give an inch. I would not, and I did not, sign that paper.

I entered the hospital for the biopsy just before the Fourth of July weekend. That circumstance also added to the suspense. I'd been told that the shortage of hospital beds was so acute that only by entering on Friday and holding down the bed over the weekend could I be assured of getting my biopsy performed on Monday. Nothing would be done over the holiday weekend —the hospital was virtually closed down except for the kitchen and I suspect even that was limping along at half-staff.

One way I entertained myself that bleak, endless Saturday and Sunday was by prowling the hospital corridors and counting empty beds. There were dozens of them and I couldn't help wondering if the over-the-weekend admission was a technique of the efficiency experts to increase hospital revenues.

With the help of a lot of sympathetic and supportive friends and relatives, I got through that awful weekend.

Then, finally, it was Monday and zero hour. I was given a sedative in my room, transferred to a stretcher and wheeled out into the corridor on the way to the operating room. A nurse noticed that I was wearing nail polish. That discovery brought on a commotion, because a hospital rule forbade nail polish in the operating room. Someone raced off for polish remover and began undoing my manicure right there in the corridor.

One of my hands had just been done when another nurse appeared and announced that the no-polish rule had recently been rescinded. Polish was now permitted. The first nurse started to cap the remover bottle and walk away. But I protested. "I'm not going in there like this," I said, waving the shiny, red-tipped fingers of one hand and the naked ones of the other. I made such a fuss that the nurse had to complete her removal job.

That's the kind of silly thing you do when you don't want to think about what's really wrong.

The biopsy was positive. The lump in my breast was cancerous. The biopsied tissue was examined by another pathologist. There was no mistake.

At first I was overcome with disbelief. Then resignation set in. Jean, I told myself, there's not a thing you can do. So let's put on a good show. Let's be brave and strong. Let's smile— and smile.

I stayed on in the hospital for two days—two very rough days—and again went up to the operating room, this time without any diversion over nail polish. On the way up, a young nurse's aide saw my grief and came over to comfort me. She gently brushed away my tears and leaned over to tell me that everything would be all right, that I would be all right. Her words of comfort fell on deaf ears. I was filled with terror. The brave façade had been just that—a façade.

Dr. Venet performed a modified radical mastectomy, meaning that he removed the breast and a number of lymph nodes from the axilla, or underarm area. He left the underlying muscle intact, and by doing this he saved me from being disfigured by the deep cavity just below the shoulder which results from removal of the pectoral muscle. (The operation that removes breast, lymph nodes and muscle is called a radical mastectomy. The operation that cuts away only the breast tissue is known as a simple mastectomy. The operation that scoops out the breast tissue but leaves the skin and nipple intact is called a subcutaneous mastectomy.)

Again relatives and friends showered me with attention—cards, flowers, visits. My father came to see me, resuming a relationship that had been almost nonexistent since my parents' divorce when I was a very small child. He brought me a stuffed teddy bear. I laughingly told my sister Gloria on the telephone, "Papa was here and he wants to pick up where he left off when I was three. But he'd better hurry up and get me through Tinkertoys and hockey sticks. I have to accelerate our relationship."

My mother came, bravely concealing her grief from me. At the hospital my mother and father met on common ground for the first time in nearly fifty years.

Dr. Venet arrived with an optimistic report. There was no involvement of the lymph nodes under the arm, and that was a very good sign. The lesion itself was only about two centimeters in size and it had all been removed. So the prognosis for a disease-free recovery was good.

My first night out of the hospital I attended a performance

of the Moiseyev Dance Company at the Metropolitan Opera House with Paul and Michael, my two grown sons. I felt very fit, strong, in touch with the world, and I was sure I could lick it.

In fact, people were commenting favorably on the cool, rational way I handled the situation. I was praised for my bravery and maturity in adjusting to the loss of my breast. Jules was pleased that I had adopted his philosophy of quiet acceptance. My son Paul, then twenty-three, and already a connoisseur of such things, told me that he had met women with very large breasts who were not at all feminine and that I was very much of a woman and would always remain so, with or without breasts.

On the outside, in this postoperative period, I appeared the picture of strength. I neither complained nor acted sorry for myself. I was friendly, hopeful and looking forward to resuming my normal activities.

But inside, there were stirrings of discontent not yet ready to surface. I guess I was sort of numb at the beginning. I liked all the attention I was getting and thought it important to maintain an image of strength and independence. As far as I knew, there wasn't anything that could be done about the fact that my breast was gone and I had always believed in making the best of things.

Besides, no one but my relatives and close friends had to know about my disfigurement. I acquired a prosthesis to wear in public—a shaped envelope of silicone that was filled with a saline solution. It adhered gently to the skin under my bra and did not have to be inserted into a pocket in the bra. I simply wore the bra over it. Everywhere I went I wore the prosthesis. It looked realistic, gave me little or no trouble and provided a satisfactory silhouette under my clothes.

Two months after the mastectomy things were going so well —at least on the surface—that my husband and I decided to go abroad for a vacation. One sunny day, while riding in a bus through the beautiful Irish countryside, the truth suddenly broke through. I thought, my God, what's happened to me?

My breast is gone forever and my body is disfigured . . . It's horrible. I wanted to scream but didn't because that isn't the way I handle deep emotions. I remembered a friend of mine, who had had both breasts removed, telling me that the first time she looked at herself, she turned on the shower and screamed at the top of her lungs for twenty minutes. I understood exactly how she felt.

From that day on I knew that I could no longer pretend to myself that everything was all right. Two things were very wrong.

First, I had been hit by cancer. But the idea of cancer is so intangible and unspecific that it is hard to grasp fully.

The other thing wrong was the loss of a breast. That I grasped very easily. In fact, ever since the operation the only way I could look at myself directly in the mirror was by raising a hand over my scar to shut it out of my vision and out of my mind. If the doorbell rang unexpectedly, I always had to check my chest to make sure I was properly put together. I was awkward and self-conscious in bed. Added to the physical embarrassment was a more subtle, psychic disturbance that I couldn't quite define, even to myself. It wasn't until some years later that I could put that malaise into words, and they wouldn't be my words. In her extraordinary book *Diary of a Pigeon Watcher*, Doris Schwerin talks about her state of mind in the year following her mastectomy. She says at one point, "There would be no more that feeling of being perfect when I loved."

I knew exactly what she meant.

Conversation

GERTRUDE

Gertrude is a dramatically attractive woman in her late forties, divorced, mother of a twenty-two-year-old son. She has an executive job in the fashion industry.

What was your first reaction to your mastectomy?
The first or the second? You know, I had two—there was a vast difference in reaction.

Let's talk about the first.
That first time I was totally shocked. It was horrifying. It happened eight years ago, and at that time I knew nothing about any possibility of reconstruction. So it was the end of the world—the end of everything. I wasn't sure before going to the operating room that I would have the breast removed. As a matter of fact, the prognosis was very good. So you can imagine how shocking it was to wake up and find I had lost a breast. All I can tell you is that it was absolutely horrifying. Eventually I adjusted somewhat—but at the beginning it was awful.

Did you have a man in your life at that time?
I had a man in my life who really didn't belong to me. I must say that he helped pull me through that terrible time. He came to the hospital every day and showed me that I was still attractive, that the surgery never made any difference to him. But then, of course, it didn't have to make any difference to him because he was married to someone else. He did not have to be that deeply involved in my problem.

In the years after my mastectomy, I discovered an interesting pattern. I found that married men seem to be more accepting of my condition than single men. Perhaps single men have more to lose, more to risk, and for that reason they are often less accepting.

Do you think married men are kinder?
Yes, they are. Simply because they can afford to be. Since they don't have to get involved on a permanent basis, they are more tolerant. No matter how deep the emotional involvement is—and I've always had long-standing relationships; the one that was going on at the time was an eight-year-old relationship—these married men really are not faced with the same risk as a single man. If I have been rejected by anyone, it's usually been by a single man.

By "rejected" you mean . . . ?
I mean that he turned away when he learned about my mastectomy. Of course, each time I met a new man I found attractive, and vice versa, I had to go through agony. How was I going to tell him? How and when was he going to notice it? How was he going to react? How should I act? I have gone through all kinds of procedures, from being completely hysterical, crying and becoming very dramatic about it, to trying to be calm, casual, even a little witty.

You're speaking about before going to bed with the man?
Yes.

When you've gone to bed with a man and you've prepared him beforehand, do you think he was deeply affected by the way you look? Did it turn him off?
In one case I think it did. This man was very fond of me, but he couldn't function. Of course, he might have had this problem anyway. But since I was very sensitive about my lost breast, I attributed his difficulty to me and what he saw when he looked at me.

Do you think that your attitude about yourself has something to do with how the man receives you sexually?
Yes, to a certain extent, but not completely. After all, it is not unusual for people to be turned off by the sight of an amputation.

If you come to him with the attitude, I'll allow you to share my body, but it's very imperfect, I'm really quite unattractive, what happens?
I can't say for sure, but I can say that hysterics and drama don't work. A projection of security, even if it's false or pretended, a take-it-or-leave-it attitude, seems to work better. But it's always hard.

I always felt constrained after I lost my breast. I never had any freedom of movement because instead of concentrating on sex itself, I had to concentrate on "Do I wear a bra or don't I wear a bra? How do I position myself? Do I take the one breast out? It was always a mess.

How did your family react to your mastectomy?
Again we are still talking about my first operation. My father was dead by then. Let me give you a bit of the background. My parents were incompatible in many respects and I have a feeling that my mother did not have any sex with my father since 1940. She had always been prudish, but she had become even more so as the years went by.

Prior to my first mastectomy I had been divorced for quite a few years. My mother always worried about my morals. She seemed uneasy whenever I had a date. She seemed to impart a feeling to me that I was committing an immoral act by going out with a man, and that I was a very "bad" mother because at the time of my divorce my son was only five years old. When I lost my breast nine years later she seemed to be relieved. She felt that perhaps this would prevent me from being interested in men (it didn't).

My mother even went so far as to insinuate to me that I should be careful about having sex because she believed that sexual intercourse could reactivate the cancer. You can see that she believed in punishment, and obviously I had to be punished —and punished.

You're saying that your moral fiber was more important to her than anything else.
Yes, that's it exactly.

Is she religious?
No, absolutely not.

What was your son's reaction?
My son never knew—at that time he was going through emotional problems of his own. I didn't want to upset him with my problem. Also, he was a young boy and I didn't want him to say inadvertently to someone, "You know, my mommy lost her breast."

You were keeping it a secret?
To some extent, yes. I did tell my son I was in the hospital and I said something about some lymph disease. He didn't ask too many questions. At fourteen he wasn't all that curious. My close friends knew about the operation, but most people didn't.

When did you first learn about reconstruction?
Each time I saw the doctor who had operated on my first breast seven years ago, I asked him, "Doctor, can anything be done?" Usually he just growled at me. But one day he said, "All right, if you insist, I'll give you the name of a plastic surgeon." I remember he was standing in the doorway of the examining room. I was still undressed and attempting to hold up my remaining breast, which had gotten rather pendulous. He looked at me and said, "But I want you to know it's not going to look like what you're holding in your hand right now."

He had a very nice nurse, and as I was leaving I said to her, "What do you know about plastic surgery?"

She said, "Well, it doesn't look very good."

The doctor cut in: "And sometimes it gets infected and you have to remove it."

The nurse said, "Yes, but people do it. You're talking about a little falsie under the skin, right?"

I said, "I guess so."

Then she said, "It really isn't very good because then you have to wear another falsie in your bra over the new little breast to compensate for the other big breast."

So of course I stopped asking. It never occurred to me that reconstruction, good reconstruction, was available. I only wish I'd known before because it might have saved—well, not my life, but a great deal of agony. Because if a doctor had started poking into the other breast to modify it, perhaps he might have found earlier that something was wrong.

What happened with the other breast?

Now we are talking about a totally different phase in my life (the black period). In February 1977 I discovered a lump in my other breast. On March second I saw a surgeon, not the one who had operated on me earlier. At that point I was ready to commit suicide. I didn't think I was able to take it, I didn't want to go on. And then he said to me, "Oh, but don't worry, we'll do a reconstruction."

I said, "But I can't. Look, there's too little skin and some of the muscle is gone all this time." (I guess I was under the impression that I had a radical.)

He said, "No, there's plenty of skin and you didn't have a radical. Besides, you're better off with two breasts removed because you don't have to adjust the real breast to match the false one."

Well, this gave me a new lease on life. I said, "All right, I want to see a plastic surgeon immediately." He gave me a name. In the meantime I dug out *The New York Times* article on reconstruction which, for an unexplainable reason, I had cut out and saved some months prior to my second mastectomy. I did research on reconstruction. I found out all there was to know.

When I went to have the second breast removed, I was the first patient scheduled for surgery that morning. I couldn't wait for the operation to be over. My mood was altogether different from the first time around. Actually I looked forward to having the breast operation. It had become large and pendulous. Now, I thought, maybe this is my opportunity to have two nice breasts. Things will be better after this.

I remember when you came to see me the first time and showed me your mastectomy scar you said, "Look at my other breast, it never was a beautiful breast anyway."

As a matter of fact, I never had beautiful breasts. I'll tell you something strange. I always had to hide my breasts. They were pear-shaped when I was a young girl and they sank very quickly. I've always been self-conscious about them. Now that I know about reconstruction, I wish that many years ago someone had told me that I could have subcutaneous plastic surgery—you know, remove all but the skin and insert an implant.

So you were planning on reconstruction after the second mastectomy and you had your nipple banked at that time. Is that why the second one was so different?

Yes, that's it exactly. I hate to be dramatic, but it was the difference between life and death. I could face the loss so much more easily the second time because I knew there were avenues open to me.

Gertrude, in one of our telephone conversations you said something that really reached me. You said, "I'm considered a sexy woman and now I feel like such a fraud." What did you really mean by that?

Let me put it this way. I guess I can say I've always projected an image of femininity and voluptuousness when I walked into a room. I've always carried a few extra pounds of pulchritude distributed in noticeable places. Now, to bridge the gap between this very vivid first impression and the disfigured reality underneath became more difficult for me than it would be for a woman who is, say, skinny or plain . . .

Yes, you raise all those expectations. So you haven't really had a relaxed relationship since your first mastectomy.
No, I have not. Except for the preexisting ongoing relationship I mentioned before. The physical aspect of the relationship gradually petered out about two years after the surgery—merely because we both had other interests. But we continued being good friends. I thought he was the most admirable, ethical, socially conscious person I ever met. After my second mastectomy he simply vanished.

The first mastectomy did not interfere with the relationship?
No, not at all. We were together one year before it happened and seven years after.

What are your plans for reconstruction?
I had the nipple from the second breast banked.* The areola is quite large, so there is the possibility the surgeon will be able to use it for both breasts.

Unfortunately, I'm still undergoing some chemotherapy at this time. But as soon as it's over and my doctor gives me a go-ahead, I'll have reconstruction.

By the way, I should tell you that my family is so frightened at the idea of reconstruction that it makes me think maybe my mother is relieved that I lost my second breast. To her, this makes me completely safe from the outside world. She was terribly upset when she heard I had reconstruction in mind. It

---

*During the mastectomy, the preserved nipple is kept on a sterile saline sponge and carefully checked by the pathologist to make sure it contains no trace of malignancy. If it passes all tests, it is temporarily implanted in the groin or abdominal area for later removal to its permanent site. A few surgeons literally put the nipple in a deep-freeze and retrieve it later.

was only when she found out that my lymph nodes were involved and that my life was in danger that she became charitable and said, "Don't worry, it's not so bad. You'll have reconstruction." She even offered me her nipples. But then the other day she said, "You know, when I think of your going under anesthesia again for the third time . . . I get the shivers."

With reconstruction, what improvement do you expect in your sex life?
It would be nice to be spontaneous in a relationship again. I don't remember what it feels like any more. In the past, when I had two breasts, I never bothered wearing plunging necklines. Now I think I would. If my reconstruction comes out the way yours did, I think I'll go crazy. I'll show it off, I'll let everyone know.

What I'm getting from you is that going through a second mastectomy, having a nodal involvement, getting chemotherapy, with all that, what's keeping you going is the promise of reconstruction—of having two breasts again.
Definitely, no question about that.

2

My Search for Reconstruction

I was angry at nature for giving me cancer, at my doctor for cutting off my breast, at society for placing so much emphasis on female breasts, at my family and friends for forcing me to mask my feelings of anger and to pretend that nothing very much had happened to me.

While I was growing up, I had liked and enjoyed my body. I did the things that young girls do: I looked at myself with admiration and found my body very pretty.

My two sons, in their early twenties at the time of my operation, had always indicated that I was rather good-looking —for a mother. My husband made it very clear that my mastectomy made no difference to him in his attitude to me. As far as he was concerned, it was just one of those sad things that happen in a lifetime. Once he was reassured that I would recover, he wanted to put the whole thing behind us.

"I'm not a youngster any more," Jules reminded me at one point. "I'm not a kid swept up in the bosom craze. You're the same woman you've always been. You are very attractive to me. And we're going on together as we always have."

I recall one night I was feeling weepy and very sorry for myself. "I think I'm going to die," I told Jules mournfully.

"Okay, if that's what you're going to do," he said. "But first let's go to the movies."

Of course I had to laugh. In his own special way he had jolted me out of my depressed mood.

Another time I was so furious at his calm that I began to throw all sorts of verbal stuff at him. He stopped me in the middle of a tirade by saying reasonably, "I'll gladly have hysterics for you, Jean, but first you'll have to tell me how that will help the situation."

I wasn't able to find *anything* that would help the situation. The upper part of my body had lost its symmetry. The skin on the flattened side where the breast had been lay tight against the ribs and chest wall. An ugly red scar stretched diagonally from my left armpit to the upper abdomen and well past the centerline of my body. With the breast missing, the area over my diaphragm had assumed an unattractive prominence.

My dissatisfaction with myself deepened as the weeks and months passed. Then somewhere, somehow, in the early 1970s I got wind of the idea of breast reconstruction. I asked Dr. Venet, a man of great sensitivity, about reconstruction. I asked him again and again. Each time he told me to forget it. For the time being. At that point, reconstruction after modified mastectomy was in its early stage; it needed the test of time and a check on worldwide results. He told me he had seen those rebuilt breasts and they weren't yet too good. I would not get the results I wanted.

While I knew he was entirely sympathetic to my sense of deprivation and to my longing to have my body look the way it had before the cruel but lifesaving amputation, it was obvious that what really concerned him was the lifesaving. I had come through a cancer operation with great success and now had every expectation of a long and useful life. Why should I want to take the risk of stirring things up?

At that time any additional surgery in an area where a malignancy had previously been found could be considered a potential health hazard. What's more, I was told, the few implant operations that had been attempted had proven esthetically less than satisfactory.

I learned later that the reconstructions Dr. Venet had seen

were those done following radical mastectomies. The extensive plastic surgery needed to create a breast and fill in the hollow areas near the shoulder and under the arm were exhausting to the patient and not much to look at, even after all the effort and trouble.

I also learned later that at the time of my surgery, the summer of 1970, the radical mastectomy, known as the Halsted operation, was the standard treatment for breast cancer. The less disfiguring modified radical was still frowned upon by most cancer surgeons. Dr. Venet was one of the relatively few surgeons who were performing the modified radical where possible. Because the operation was new, it needed the test of time to show it would give results as good as the standard radical's. Dr. Venet still felt concern about a possible recurrence of the cancer. So no wonder he was opposed to complicating the picture by allowing me to undertake something as then untried as a breast reconstruction. He was stalling me for my own sake.

That's why every time I mentioned the subject of replacement, this good doctor firmly rejected the idea temporarily and urged that I make the best of my situation by using a breast prosthesis inside my bra and by focusing on the fact that I was an attractive, healthy woman.

That's what he told me back then. Today his attitude is somewhat different. Reassured by the success, from the medical point of view, of thousands of skillfully performed reconstructions, he now feels the procedure is safe enough to approve for some of his patients. In some instances he outlines the possibility of reconstruction at the same time he breaks the bad news of the need for biopsy. He does this because he has seen many successful reconstructions as well as the joyous relief of patients who have had their longings for a new breast brought to a happy reality. My reconstruction was one of the first of these.

Today this same surgeon says to those of his mastectomy patients he considers to be suitable candidates that they should know, if interested, that they can probably have a breast reconstruction in a year or possibly less, that a plastic surgeon can build a new breast after the old, diseased one is removed and that even a new nipple can be built.

At any rate, back in that dark time, the early 1970s, I got no help from my doctor. And whenever I began to talk to Jules about reconstruction, I got no reaction at all. He was completely indifferent to the thought. He could see no need for searching out a way to change the inevitable. He was willing to live with what had happened, and he thought I should make my peace with my changed body and learn to accept it.

That, however, was not my point of view. I was always achingly aware of the change, the loss. I even became squeamish. The sight of blood now brought on shakes and shivers, although back at college I'd been the coolest frog-cutter in the physiology lab.

I remember that the first movie I saw after my operation was Z, a tense story of espionage and torture in Fascist Greece. Some of the scenes were so excruciatingly painful to me that several times I ran from my seat crying and had to spend time in the ladies' room composing myself.

Every day, when I put on my clothes and took them off I saw the scarring, the lost breast, the ugly reminder of cancer. I hated the mutilation so much that I no longer liked myself.

That was the real problem—the increasing self-hate that grew out of my sense of being incomplete. No matter what was happening, I had a gnawing feeling of dissatisfaction with myself, a sinking sensation of unhappiness that this was going to be me from here on in. For the rest of my life I would have to put up with a mutilated body. And from the very depths of myself I loathed the idea.

One day I picked up a copy of *Vogue* magazine and read an article by a writer named Simona Morini about a plastic surgeon in Switzerland who was doing breast reconstructions.

Quickly and eagerly I tore out the article and rushed to my doctor. "What about the work this man is doing in Switzerland?" I asked him. "What do you think?"

He didn't think I ought to try anything like that. He thought it too new—too unproven. He didn't want me to take any chances. He wanted me to wait a bit more.

Of course I didn't want to take chances. I didn't want to do anything rash, but two years had passed since my operation and I was still grieving over my loss.

A short time later I heard about a plastic surgeon at a major New York hospital who was doing breast reconstructions. I called him immediately and made an appointment. After examining the scarred area carefully, he offered his opinion: "Yes, there's enough skin to work with. I can do the job. But what the hell are you waiting for? If you want to look like a *Playboy* centerfold, you'd better hurry up—you're nearly fifty years old."

I ran from his office shaking. Here, at last, was a surgeon who held out the possibility of restoration, but I couldn't handle his insensitivity and vulgarity. He hadn't the slightest feeling of what it was like to be a woman with a breast missing. He thought all I wanted was to become a sex symbol. That wasn't it at all. I just wanted to be back where I'd started from—a woman, whole, intact.

Again I put my search aside. Then in 1973 I went to see a dermatologist about a routine skin problem totally unrelated to my original cancer. She was a woman, very lovely, fresh and young, still in her early thirties. When I stripped for her, she saw the prosthesis in my bra. "Why don't you do something about that?" she asked me.

"Like what?"

"You don't have to look like that," she said. "You can have that breast restored. There are plastic surgeons who are doing that work. I've seen it in the clinic. The results are really pretty good."

She gave me this information with such simplicity and honesty that I believed her right away. I was so excited, I reached out and hugged her. A feeling of exhilaration that I had not known for a long time surged through my body.

She wrote down the name of Dr. Saul Hoffman. As I left her office I felt a marvelous new hope stirring within me. It wasn't just that she had given me a plastic surgeon's name. It was her whole attitude: she was concerned, both as a woman and a doctor, that I was not whole and that I wanted to be. My longing to be restored seemed entirely natural to her. No speeches, no scoldings, no cautions. Instead, concern and caring. I felt I was on my way.

3

The Start of My Reconstruction

Dr. Saul Hoffman is a small man, very gentle, soft-spoken, without a silky bedside style but with a quiet way about him that conveys great sincerity. He examined me and nodded his head in a very positive manner. "Yes, you're a good candidate for reconstruction," he said. "You had a modified radical mastectomy, so that means that your pectoral muscle is intact. You didn't have radiation. There's enough skin. Everything looks favorable."

He explained to me that the tight skin on my left side could be separated from the chest wall so as to form a pocket and a silicone prosthesis placed in the pocket.

I asked him just what silicone is, and he described it as an inert substance that has the marvelous property of not being rejected by the body. Because the body accepts it as if it were natural tissue, it is used in a variety of ways by plastic surgeons and other doctors. In a fairly stiff form, it serves as a temporary or permanent replacement for cartilage. In a form that is rather like rubber it can be shaped into a round or oval envelope that can be filled with more silicone of a jellylike consistency or with a saline solution. This silicone envelope is then inserted under the breast tissue to enlarge a too small breast or placed under the skin and the old mastectomy scar to rebuild a breast lost to cancer.

He also explained that silicone in a quite different form is used to make the outer casing of cardiac pacemakers that are introduced under the skin to regulate malfunctioning hearts. Hundreds of thousands of these silicone-enclosed pacemakers are in use and have been for many years—attesting to the safety of this material inside the body.

I asked Dr. Hoffman how many breast restorations he'd done. His answer wasn't very specific. I asked him if I could meet some patients he'd operated on. From his reply I sensed that he'd done only a handful of reconstructions, but that he and his patients were happy with the results.

He showed me one or two photographs, before and after. In the after ones, taken immediately after surgery, the skin looked raw and scarred, the stitches showed and the results weren't especially attractive. I realize now that surgeons deliberately show you postoperative photographs that leave a good deal to be desired. They don't want to promise you too much. They want you to prepare yourself to accept modest improvement.

As it happened, the unappetizing aspect of those photos didn't bother me a bit. All I saw was the second breast, miraculously put back where it belonged. Nothing else registered in my mind. Only the breast, back in place.

What I liked best about Dr. Hoffman was his empathy for women. He spoke disapprovingly of the way some surgeons had been doing radical mastectomies when lesser surgery could have been used. He was upset by the cancer surgeons' lack of concern for the patient's psyche. I had the feeling that because he was a plastic surgeon he understood women better than regular surgeons did. He could see beyond the incision, into the scarring on the personality.

On that first visit Dr. Hoffman showed me a breast implant and explained the various types. The one he gave me to hold was a strange thing to touch. It was a kind of self-contained gelatinous mass. Very soft and shapeless with a silicone exterior that gave it form and a silicone gel inside. It had the consistency of a breast in a very loose way. The doctor explained that once it's in place, the skin provides contour and rigidity. He showed me another type that is filled with a saline solution after it is placed under the skin.

He further explained that because of the tightness of the skin over my ribs the implant would have to be positioned high on the chest wall. That meant the implant would be both higher and rounder than my own right breast which had acquired, with time, a slight droop. I've always worn a size 36B bra and my breast size was well balanced with my height of five feet, seven and a half inches.

Dr. Hoffman went on to tell me that sometimes it is necessary to do a second operation in order to match the remaining natural breast to the newly implanted one. That upset me very much. I was strongly opposed to any cutting into my good breast. I was very concerned about the sensitivity of the remaining nipple—I didn't want to lose that under any circumstances. "Now wait a minute," I objected, "I don't want any surgery on my good breast."

The doctor seemed not to hear me. "We'll see what happens," he said. "We'll wait—maybe you won't need anything done."

He explained that he could not decide on the exact size and shape of the implant until I was in the operating room. The final decision among various sizes and types would be made in the course of surgery when he could determine just what size pocket was possible. Without promising me anything one way or the other, he let the hope hang in the air that the match between the implant and the real thing would be close enough to avoid further surgery. I let it go at that. I would handle this whole thing one step at a time.

I made up my mind immediately to go ahead. In my initial enthusiasm, I began to talk to my friends. I found out right away that that was a mistake. The negative responses of my family and friends to my decision to have reconstruction made the interval of waiting a very sad period in my life. Nobody seemed to understand why I looked forward to this operation with so much joy. My friends couldn't make sense out of what

I was doing. Breast reconstruction was totally unheard of at that time, so, of course, it sounded risky and rash. Everyone tried in all kinds of ways to discourage me. But the greatest sting was the statement from an old friend: "Jean, I had no idea you were so vain."

It was like a slap on the face. Was it vanity? I asked myself. Was I inane, silly, self-involved, chasing after my lost youth? What was I trying to prove?

I settled into a period of intense self-examination. I searched out my feelings and my motives. I tried to be ruthlessly honest with myself.

No, it wasn't like a face-lift. I wasn't trying to roll back the clock. I wasn't out to make myself sexy and desirable. My husband was entirely satisfied with the one-sided me. Even in his understated way he had made that perfectly clear in words, actions and attitude.

I was the one who was dissatisfied, still angry and rebellious at the mutilation of my body, still aching with incompleteness. Most of the time, of course, I hid that ache. Over the years I had learned to push the dissatisfaction to the back of my mind. I kept it tucked away there as I went on with my life. I functioned very well as a person. There was no question—I could go on that way indefinitely if it was necessary.

But the whole point was that it really wasn't necessary—not any more. Something better, much better, was right at hand, easily available. All I wanted to do was to get back where I started, look the way I had once looked. The opportunity was right there and that's why I was going ahead.

One disturbing comment came from a friend who was deeply concerned about my health. She told me, "You must be crazy to let them go in there and poke around among those old cells. How do you know you won't touch off another cancer?"

I went back to Dr. Venet, who had performed the mastectomy and had discouraged all my earlier inquiries. This time, to my total delight, he did not try to stop me.

"Yes, by all means do it," he told me. "You've had a three-

and-a-half-year interval between the initial surgery and this reconstruction. That's ample time for healing. The new techniques are very good. I think you should be pleased with the results."

Why the about-face? Time, greater knowledge, more experience with implants, sharper awareness of the sense of deprivation felt by mastectomy patients—all these factors had persuaded Dr. Venet and many of his colleagues with equally conservative views that reconstruction was both safe and desirable.

In addition, the climate had changed dramatically. Many more patients were having the modified radical mastectomies that lend themselves more easily to reconstruction. Cancer was coming out of the closet. Self-examination and mammography were contributing to earlier detection.

Dr. Venet gave me his blessing and sent the pathology report made at the time of the mastectomy to Dr. Hoffman so that the plastic surgeon would have a full record of my case.

As for my husband, Jules said, "I know you've made up your mind, so go ahead. I don't see the necessity for what you're putting yourself through. But if you think it will make it easier for you to live with yourself, all right—it's your body."

So what it really boiled down to was that I was alone, as I had been when I first began the search for a plastic surgeon. Even if I could make contact with someone because of my despair, who would have the answer, who would speak the words that would dispel the heavy cloud hanging over my life? No one had the technical expertise to say, "Do this, it is good for you. Avoid this, it will harm you."

How marvelous it would have been if everyone who knew me could have joined hands around me in a warm, loving circle to assure me that they understood what I was feeling and to tell me again and again that they shared my excitement and anticipation over the extraordinary step I was about to take—the reconstruction of my breast.

I didn't get that reaction. Maybe it was unrealistic of me to expect that anyone else could grasp the depth of my feeling of loss and my soaring expectations of recovery. I was out there in deep water entirely on my own.

I was facing more surgery, more anesthesia, another hospital stay, with all the accompanying risks, because reconstruction was something I was doing for myself, not for anybody else. Just for *me*.

My first visit to Dr. Hoffman was in January 1974. After assuring me that he knew how deprived I felt with just one breast, he went on to say that in about ten years he expected reconstruction to become so much the norm that cancer surgeons would be making, where possible, certain adjustments in their operations to facilitate later reconstruction.

Dr. Hoffman was wrong by about seven years. In less than three years more cancer surgeons, while still putting their primary emphasis on eradication of the cancer, were already tailoring their operations in certain ways to the needs of subsequent rebuilding. A few were even permitting the plastic surgeon to be present at the mastectomy and in appropriate cases to temporarily attach the nipple of the amputated breast to the thigh or groin for later use.

My reconstruction was done in February 1974 on the same floor of the same hospital where the mastectomy had been performed. I was in the hospital for five days. I had some discomfort the first few days, but it was easily bearable. In a way it was like the discomfort of having a baby: though the pain was much, much less, the psychology was the same. You know you're in the hospital for a positive, constructive reason and you are looking forward to the results with eager anticipation instead of the dread of awaiting the results of a biopsy. Any pain is forgotten the minute it's over.

I found once again the same nurse's aide who had sat and wept with me three and a half years earlier as I was being taken up to surgery. What a lovely reunion! And when I told her why

I was in the hospital this time, she could hardly believe her ears. She'd never heard of such a procedure. She walked out of the room shaking her head in wonder at this surgical phenomenon of restoring what had once been removed—presumably forever.

Conversation

ELIZABETH

Elizabeth is married, lives in the Midwest, has two children in their twenties and had undergone mastectomy less than a month before our conversation.

Elizabeth, what response do you get when you talk about reconstruction?
My husband is supportive. But then I really haven't given him a chance to be anything else because I'm the one who really wants it. I've found that in my situation the shock was a little more devastating because of the way it happened. Normally, if a woman discovers a lump, and has to find a doctor and make an appointment and then wait for that appointment, then go to see him—at that point she is already a little bit psyched. She's already worrying, My God, what will happen to me?
In my case, I was lying on my hospital bed at nine-fifteen in the evening, ready to go for a hysterectomy because of fibroids the next morning at seven-thirty. I'd been prepped, everything had been done, and my doctor came in sort of routinely, night-before-the-operation, and said casually, "Let me give you an examination."
He did the right breast first, then leaned over and did the left. And I saw his expression change. I said, "Now wait a minute. You're not a very good actor. You've just noticed something. You'd better tell me what it is."
His expression was a give-away of the fact that he was concerned. What he was concerned about was a lump he had just found. There were two surgeons in town, either of whom he thought should look at me. "One of them," he told me, "goes to bed very early and maybe I can get him here at five in the

morning." He was still thinking of that seven-thirty operation time. The other one was out for the evening, but he lived fairly close to the hospital and there was a chance he could get there later.

Meanwhile I called my husband, but it was too late for him to come to the hospital—visiting hours were over. About eleven-forty-five that night Dr. G. walked into my room. He examined me and he didn't like what he found. He suggested that since I had the operating room for seven-thirty, he should do a biopsy. He promised that he would do nothing but the biopsy because I was not going into that operating room not knowing what I was going to lose—a uterus, a breast or just a little bit of tissue to be examined.

He also explained to me the various possibilities if the breast was malignant. He told me about a treatment available in Boston with x-rays. He told me about plastic surgery and about banking the nipple. He gave me a rather concise picture of the various possibilities.

When I came out of surgery, I knew there was a malignancy. I made up my mind that I was going to look into all the possibilities of what could be done. All I knew was that there had never been cancer in my family. I had never taken the birth control pill. I don't smoke. I don't eat an excessive amount of meat.

The first thing I wanted was another pathology report. I went to a leading breast clinic in Chicago, and a doctor there looked at the biopsy. He said, "The sooner the better, the sooner the better." Everyone said that I should have a mastectomy immediately.

But I still wasn't prepared for it in my head. I explored the possibility of a lumpectomy. I'm glad now I didn't opt for that. I don't think I would have really felt secure. I looked into a procedure that involves intensive bombardment of the lesion area with radiation. It's done five days a week for six weeks. The people who do it in Boston feel their rate of cure is as high as the surgical procedure's. When I talked to them, they'd handled a hundred and thirty-nine cases. They thought mine was suitable. My husband was very doubtful about it. He preferred going with a sure, proven thing.

We have a close friend who is a doctor and he said to me, "I want you to see an oncologist. An oncologist is not in the business of any particular treatment. He's in the business of evaluating tumors."

So I made an appointment with an oncologist, a very pleasant older gentleman. I wonder whether the advice I got would have been the same if he had been a younger man. He did an examination and a reevaluation of the pathology report. He sat down with the x-ray people who do that six-week procedure and left word for me to call him at home that night. When I phoned him, he said, "I don't think you have the time."

So I went ahead and had the mastectomy.

At that time you knew that reconstruction was available, didn't you?

Yes, and I'll tell you frankly that if it hadn't been dangled in front of me, I might not have made the decision to go ahead. I might have pushed for a little more investigation. I'd heard of a woman doctor in Canada who's been successfully doing radiation without surgery for thirty years. I might have gone to see her to find out if she could save the breast. But everyone was screaming at me, "You've got to do it right away." You see, the thing had grown so fast from January, when my doctor had noticed only a slight thickening, to mid-March, when he found a real lump. That's why everyone was frantic for me to have it done.

Afterwards, when they found nothing else in any tissue and all the nodes were okay, I realized I might have taken more time. But it was too late. The breast was gone.

You know, I never thought about death at all. I didn't think of dying. I thought of the illness that I had and the different ways to cure it. But I never looked death in the face. I felt so alive that the fear of dying never came into my decision.

How did you feel after the mastectomy?
I felt ugly. No matter what reassurance I got that I was the same person, whether it was from my husband or from other people, if I was that way in their eyes—fine, wonderful for them. But not for me. And I have to live with me. I look down, I look to the side, but I can't stand in front of a mirror and look at myself. I don't even make any effort. Why should I put myself through it if reconstruction is in the offing?

I had a discussion with the same doctor friend who advised me earlier about the surgery. He is terribly upset with me. He feels I'm much too intense about the whole thing, that my search for plastic surgery is ridiculous. He thinks I should get adjusted to the situation, and maybe in a year's time if I still feel the same way, then go ahead. But I said to him, "Why? What do I have to prove by adjusting to this? I don't want to go into plastic surgery with as little, hurriedly collected knowledge as I had when I went into the original surgery."

I feel there's a lot of male chauvinism in the attitude of doctors. They seem to be saying that if you need your left breast to feel sexy, there's something wrong with you. I tell them it's not that at all. I just like having a left breast better than not having it.

How were you affected sexually after the surgery?
It was hard because I couldn't let anyone come that close. I still go to bed with a bra and a prosthesis on. I feel more comfortable that way. I'll drop one side. But I'm vulnerable, so vulnerable that I don't need someone saying to me that it doesn't matter. Because it isn't what matters to them—it's what matters to me. I slept in a black bra last night and playfully asked my husband how it felt to be in bed with Moishe Dayan when I lowered my bra strap.

I think one reason there is so much misunderstanding is that the whole sexual experience has to do with self-love. And how can you love yourself when you have an amputation?

How does your husband feel toward reconstruction?
He's terribly supportive. I have a twenty-three-year-old son and a twenty-one-year-old daughter. We play no games with them. I laid it all on the line for them. My daughter is heading into pre-med, so she went out and asked the people she knows a lot of questions. My son is very sensitive and attuned to emotions, and on his own did a lot of looking into the subject. I was very touched by this. For him to care enough to go looking for information caused me to look at him with new eyes. His sense of caring was nice to have.

My husband's mother had had a mastectomy years ago. That was one of the things that bothered me. She's always lopsided, her prosthesis is never in the right place.

Maybe if this had happened when I was younger, when my children were smaller, when being all right in my husband's eyes was my whole world—maybe then I wouldn't have bothered about reconstruction. But I've changed dramatically in the last eight or ten years of my life. I was married at nineteen, was led around by the nose. If people snapped their fingers, I'd jump.

However, with maturing, I've become my own person, not my husband's appendage. I have a great need to do something for myself, just for me, and that's what the reconstruction means to me—doing something for me. As soon as I am able to I will go ahead with reconstruction. My doctor says I have to wait six to eight months to let the breast area heal completely.

I'm very perplexed about women who do not wish this rehabilitation. I think in many cases it represents fear. I don't think enough doctors present this as a positive next step. Their attitude still is: First I remove the cancer, then you make an adjustment to the deprivation. I think this is a great influence on many women.

Then, too, there's still a certain stigma to exhibiting yourself as someone who cannot take this kind of loss calmly and stoically. People try to make you feel immature, overindulged or vain because you want to be the self you once were. I think the whole thing is really a question of being yourself. And every woman has that right.

4

My Reconstruction

This is what was done to me. An eight-inch vertical incision was made along my rib cage underneath my left arm. The incision was made in this particular place in order to interfere as little as possible with the circulation of blood in the skin over my chest. Then, under the skin on the chest a pocket was made just large enough to hold the implant in place.

After the silicone prosthesis was inserted, the opening was closed, stitched and left to heal. As surgical procedures go, this was a very simple one, for it involved no vital organs and no basic bodily functions, such as breathing or digesting. The cutting was on the surface of the body. In fact, the skin on the chest wall is the key to the operation, for it is the limiting factor and determines the size of the pocket that can be created.

One thing I want to be very clear about. The silicone prosthesis used in reconstruction should not be confused with the liquid silicone injections to inflate the breasts which were once something of a fad and have since been widely looked on with disfavor because of their adverse effects on the human body. It is generally agreed among surgeons that these injections should not be used for breast augmentation and they are never used for breast reconstruction.

What did I look like? First, a reconstructed breast without a nipple or areola is rather an odd-looking thing. It has the empty look of a dressmaker's dummy. Or you could say it resembles a cartoon drawing of a nude woman when the artist is restrained from drawing a real breast and just sketches a curve.

No matter. To me, it was fantastic. Miraculously, I had two breasts. One was high, round, virginal, just budded, and devoid of nipple. The other was lower and fuller. Picasso would have loved the way I looked. I distinctly remember a painting of his of a woman with wildly unmatched breasts. But I didn't care. There were *two* breasts—count them, two, and that's what mattered.

Almost from the moment the anesthesia wore off, I was very curious to find out about the reactions of the medical staff to the surgery that had been performed on me. Remember—at this point a breast reconstruction was still an oddity. The interns and residents, I soon found out, were only mildly curious. They seemed too swamped by their duties to pay very much attention to me and to the lesson I was trying to teach them. For already, barely out of the ether, I wanted to make them aware of reconstruction. My own feeling was that they should have shown more curiosity, since for most of them this was the first rebuilt breast in their medical experience.

The nurses showed somewhat more interest. Whenever one came into the room, I made a point of telling her exactly what had happened. I was speaking to them from a feminist's rather than a patient's point of view. I wanted them to know both for themselves and for future patients about this option that was available to breast cancer victims.

The nurse who was most interested was a very young one who laughingly called herself Patty Papsmear. She came in to give me a Pap test. Some marvelous legislation protective of women had made it mandatory in New York to offer hospital patients this test for cervical cancer. Patty was sweet and supportive and so happy to learn that women could, at last, do something to correct the deformity of a mastectomy. "Let me see what they did to you" she said. I showed her, and she was delighted at what she was sure would be important and welcome news for thousands of women.

Patty shared my joy and promised to send all the mastectomy patients on the floor to see the magical alternative to a piece of foam rubber stuffed in the bra. Patty felt both concerned for other women and personally involved, for I later learned that she had a sister who had undergone a mastectomy. At Patty's urging, one patient did come to see me. She was amazed. "My God," she said, "why didn't anybody tell me? I hope I'll be able to have this done. Why didn't I know about it?"

One day while I was still in the hospital, up and walking around, a close friend came to visit me. We walked together to the smoking room and sat on the sofa next to each other. "Vera," I said, "do you want to play a game?"

"Sure," she said.

"All right, move close to me and put your arm around me. Make believe we're . . . Well, just sort of let your fingers go along this breast and see how it feels."

Vera was a good enough friend to understand what I was getting at. We played the game. She put her arm around me, let her fingers play a bit and said, "It's very nice."

"Are you sure?" I asked.

"Yes, it's quite nice. Not bad at all."

That was what I wanted to hear. The implant was still very firm at that time. (It gradually softens as the skin stretches.) I could see it looked natural, even at this incomplete stage. Now I knew it *felt* natural.

Now, I asked myself, would I be able at last to get the monkey off my back? Would I now be able to look at all the pages of bra ads in the magazines without shuddering, watch full-bosomed women walk toward me on the street without being reminded of my deformity, put an end to my compulsive involvement with breasts and get in tune with other, more important aspects of life?

Please let it be, I thought. Let me go back to being the outward person I was before my operation. Let me be finished with the self-involvement, the fear, the feeling of a sword of Damocles hanging over my head. Let me feel complete, attractive again, not less so than all the women around me.

Of course, I knew perfectly well then, as I do now, that the essence of being female consists of many subtleties and complexities, some visible externally, some hidden deep in the psyche. Two breasts are not, by any means, the sum total of a woman's female identity. And yet the breasts are undeniably important. Their value is both utilitarian and symbolic. No question, the sexual symbolism of the breast is vastly exaggerated in our society. But scoff as we may at the cult of the breast and the worship of any given season's deep-breasted love goddess, few of us can detach ourselves from the stereotypes of our time. Take away a breast, and suddenly even the best adjusted of us is likely to feel deprived, diminished, bereft in her essential femaleness.

Then reverse that deep current of loss with the almost overnight restoration of a breast—never mind that the replacement is far from perfect—and suddenly the deprivation vanishes.

For me the change was instantaneous and almost overwhelming. After years of feeling alienated from my own body, now at last I was comfortable in it again. I no longer had to wince when I looked at myself. I was no longer spoiled, no longer less of a woman. I was almost whole again. Still lopsided, still without a nipple, but almost whole.

It's hard for me to make clear at this point that I was not concerned solely with superficial aspects of beauty. Of course, I looked a good deal better, both nude and in clothes—I couldn't help noticing that. I was glad my body was beginning to please me once again. The mirror on the back of the bathroom door, once my friend and then my enemy, was beginning to be my friend again. That in itself was no minor matter.

But beyond the small vanities of daily life, something exciting and liberating had happened to me. The only way I can describe it is to say that I was tasting again the joy of wholeness. I had finally satisfied my almost obsessive need to become intact in body. And in so doing I discovered I had set free my energies, my interests, my whole personality.

It was as if I had been released from some kind of bondage. Now I was free for living and loving. I experienced a fantastic surge of energy. I knew how a butterfly must feel when it emerges from the chrysalis. I, too, wanted to fly.

Even while I was still in the hospital I underwent this wonderful sense of awakening after a long, troubled sleep. Now it came to me that in spite of my age on the calendar, I was still in the morning of my life. The sun was out. The world was beckoning. The whole cancer experience was behind me, shelved at last, pushed out of daily consciousness. The oppressive sense of doom was lifted. Reconstruction had done this for me.

Conversation

SELMA

Selma, fifty-three, is a singer. She is from a large family, is married and the mother of two grown children.

What was your reaction when you first knew you had to have a breast removed?
When I went into the hospital I didn't really believe it was going to be serious. I didn't have a lump, only some nodes and small tissue changes and the gynecologist wanted them looked at. The mammogram wasn't conclusive. I made an appointment for a biopsy at Memorial Hospital in New York, but I didn't think I had anything serious. The worst thing was that I had to wait six weeks for a bed and had to stay by the telephone. I was very fond of my breasts and was always considered a very sexy looking woman. I had very large breasts. It was the Marilyn Monroe era and I was glad to be well endowed. But at the same time I had other things to live for besides my body. So I signed the release at the time of the biopsy.

They did not remove my breast in the operating room. They did a deep biopsy in both breasts and sent the material to pathology on Friday and had me stay in bed for the whole weekend to get the report. I didn't know until Sunday night that I had to go back into surgery.

What was your reaction after surgery?
Someone in my own family had died of another kind of cancer, and when the doctor told me he didn't have to remove the muscle and all of my glands, and after a few days he told me there was no invasion of the lymph glands and I wouldn't need postoperative therapy—it may seem funny to you, but I experienced a high. I came through smiling. I was happy to see

the sun come up. In fact, I sang in the hospital while I was still in my hospital gown. It was only the third day, my arm was still in a sling, but the doctor asked if I'd entertain some of the patients. I wasn't sure why he was doing it—whether he was testing my lungs to see if they were still functioning or what —but I said, "Of course." When I got out there and started to sing, I got another high because I realized that nothing in my outer life had changed at all. Any role I played for the outside world was the same as before. The patients and the nurses applauded and crowded around me. I was so turned on I didn't sleep for two days.

My husband and a lot of relatives came to visit me that night and when I told them that I sang that day, they just couldn't believe me.

Did you cry at all?
I never cried in the hospital. Maybe it's because part of my profession makes you a clown. I made jokes like, "You show me the man who can take two breasts in his mouth and I'll show you Joe E. Brown." And I said, "My husband's fortunate enough to have Audrey Hepburn on one side and Sophia Loren on the other. What man can say he's got two in one?" I don't know why, but a lot of humor came out of me.

What happened when you went home?
For the first few days everything was fine. I'd gotten so many flowers and cards and calls that I said, "I went to my funeral and I had a marvelous time." I never knew so many people loved me. That was great and my husband was marvelous. Of course he was very tense and concerned. He was afraid I'd feel devastated and mourn the loss of my breast. But at that moment I was concerned about relieving his tension. My mother-in-law told me that he cried, and my husband doesn't cry easily. In fact, I never saw him cry.

The first night when I was home, I suggested that he put in my diaphragm and we have sex—not so much for the sex as for the feeling of closeness and intimacy, and I wanted him to know that it hadn't changed for us, that I was not going to hide in a closet. I was still bandaged and I knew he would be very concerned about approaching me on sex that first night I was home. I think he might have been afraid he might hurt me. But when he put in my diaphragm, it was such a turn-on for him that he had a strongly emotional reaction. He was so happy to be relieved of the tension.

I had a nurse for a few days but then I said, "Steve, you'll have to assist me with my bandages. I don't want to be in the bathroom alone or take a bath by myself. I'm not crazy about looking at me, but we're going to have to get used to it." So I had him draw my bath, stay in the bathroom, wash my back, change my dressing. He became very involved in it. He would look at the scar and the stitches and say, "Gee, it doesn't really look that bad. It's not that frightening." It was almost as though he was born to be a physician.

Did you have a reaction at any point?

Well, the first reaction was not to my own illness. Don't forget, I was at Memorial Hospital, the big cancer hospital, and I was able to leave the hospital. There were several women in my room who were not going to be able to leave. Some of the others would be going back again and again. So I felt I was the healthiest person in there. Being in any other hospital among people who'd had an appendix out or had a baby, I might have been devastated. But in Memorial you have an entirely different perspective.

I became especially fond of one woman. She had cancer of the colon, and I knew she wasn't going to be able to leave the hospital. I could see the torment, the torture she was going through. I used to read to her. If she got confused at night from the morphine, I'd get out of bed and call the nurse. Helping her allowed me not to think about myself so much. She wrote me after I was home that she'd moved to my bed because she thought mine was luckier than hers.

My first reaction to the operation related to her. I developed a spastic colon. I had such a tight feeling in my stomach about her illness I couldn't stand the thought of her death. I had experienced the loss of a sister the previous year, and now I was experiencing the loss of another person of whom I had become very fond. It didn't occur to me immediately that it was my own loss I was feeling. I was operated on in November. That winter we went to St. Maarten and I bought two very nice bathing suits and I looked stunning in them. But it bothered me to think that I had to be a little more covered up than the others on the beach. Then I would see their cleavage and that's when it zeroed in on me.

The first time I went on the beach, it hit me. One man said to his wife, "Why don't you keep yourself like Selma?" I have a small body, I've always watched my diet and exercised a lot. I said to myself, "Idiot, be thankful for what you have." Then, at the hotel, when I took off my prosthesis and put it in the dresser, I thought, What if the maid sees it? And when my husband and I made love, I found I couldn't be as abandoned as I used to be. I had to approach it from a slightly different angle. I had been an aggressive person sexually, now I had to start the sexual ball rolling in a different way. I had to keep the bra on for a little bit longer. I had to get into the proper mood before I could take it off.

When did you first get interested in reconstruction?

I think it was in '71. I went to one plastic surgeon, but he handled me rather indifferently. I rather felt I was an object, not a subject. He didn't look into my eyes, didn't relate to my sensitivity. So I decided I was getting along well enough with the one breast. If he'd been a little more sensitive, I might have pursued it.

What about your original surgeon?

He was very kind about it, but at that time he'd pat me on the knee and say, "You'll have to do with one what you once did with two."

What was the attitude of men toward you?
I must say this about men. They were not put off by it. They were just as eager to approach me on a sexual basis—they would easily and gladly have accepted any sexual liaison with me, even with one breast. They thought I had no reason to be ashamed or to fear it.

I must tell you about one way-out thing I did—something I don't believe many women with breast surgery have done. I went to a nudist camp.

You really did?
Yes, I did. This was only six months after surgery. I have friends who've been nudists ever since I've known them—at least twenty years. I never wanted to go to the camp with them. My husband and I thought we'd feel too vulnerable, even though this is a family establishment, not a place for meeting and making connections. There are children there, grandparents, whole families. They're basically Europeans and health faddists.

Another friend, not a nudist, said she and her husband would like to go because the sexual revolution was coming into its own and she felt this was something she wanted to do. She asked me to introduce her to my friends who belonged to the nudist camp. I introduced the two couples and they asked me to come with them. So I decided to take a chance on myself. I prepared a very beautiful corsage of plastic flowers and I went to the nudist camp with the flowers taped on the area where the breast had been removed. I felt it was copping out to wear a bra.

Well, I astonished those people. They'd never seen or experienced anything like it. They'd never seen a person who'd had a breast removed and who'd exhibit her entire body and just put the flowers there. So I kidded them. I said, I'd made a little wreath, a little corsage, for my dear departed friend. I'm still proud of the rest of my body. I walked around that way and I was very high after I did it. I was saying, "I'm going to accept my body and the world is going to accept my body." We actually joined the nudist camp and went there for a while. There was some negative feedback. Another woman there had had a breast removed and she was upset by the fact that I walked around without a bra. She had never done it. She said it would really be more becoming if I'd wear a bra. None of the men objected. Some of the younger men were so turned on and attracted by it that had I desired a liaison, I'm sure I could have had one.

What about the second mastectomy?

There was a little hardening around the biopsy incision I'd had in the past on the remaining breast, and at first they thought it was just a little scar tissue. But as it turned out, it was the tiniest millimeter of a malignant tumor. I didn't have an invasion of the glands and I didn't need postoperative therapy, but I did have to have the second breast off. By that time, I had read in *Time* magazine about a reconstruction on a young lady in Florida. I told my surgeon that I planned to have reconstruction. I certainly didn't want to be without any breasts at all. I think on the second side the doctor left a little more tissue, a little softness on the upper part of the chest wall so it would be easier to rebuild.

How did you manage sexually with both breasts off?

I refused to hide myself. I tried going without a bra when we made love, but I think that upset my husband. It made him feel that I had been clobbered. He was so distressed, he said, "Boy, they did a job on you, kid." When he said that, I knew he couldn't take it without the bra. I slept without the bra. When we had sex I always started with the bra. So I did feel a little deprivation. But there's no activity you can't go back to—that's for sure.

My daughter was fifteen at the time of the first operation and no way was I going to traumatize her and have her think that it was a bad thing to grow up to be a woman and then have your life over if you don't have breasts. You have your intelligence, your personality, your work. What's more, you have sexual attractiveness. If you go around suffering, everyone else is going to suffer with you. Neither my son nor my daughter doubted that I could get up and go do my thing. They knew I went to the nudist camp. They didn't care to go, but they thought it was a really right-on move for me to make.

What about the reconstruction?
The plastic surgeon I went to see showed me two tiny little transplants. They hardly looked worth the effort. They were so flat and tiny I thought I wouldn't end up with more breasts than an eight-year-old child. Not that that stopped me. But he said I wasn't ready yet. I should wait a few months. But in the meantime why didn't I let him do my eyes? Now I'm all for plastic surgery and face-lift or anything—but how insensitive could he be? I'd been traumatized by a bilateral breast removal three months before, and now he was talking about taking a tuck in my eyelids. So I dropped him.

I went to a different plastic surgeon and told him how I'd wanted my breasts done and the other doctor had talked about my eyes. He said, "Your breasts, why you're a beautiful lady." He obviously misunderstood the situation and thought I wanted my breasts made bigger or smaller or whatever. Well, when he found out what I wanted, he told me that breast reconstruction was still in a new stage, still experimental.

"We're getting some results," he said, "but not the results I would like to see. I'd like you to hang in there for a few more years. One of these days they'll come up with a better operation and then you'll be a candidate."(Remember, this was 1973.)
So I waited. I lived that way for four years.

How did you fare without any breasts?
Well, I had moments of feeling badly, but on the other hand, I found a substitute for singing. I played a lot of tennis, I took three or four lessons a week. I went to the nudist camp once, but I didn't enjoy it much any more. My sex life continued pretty much as usual—I did not intend to be deprived

of the pleasure of intimacy. I still kept my bra on, but I had not lost my sexual charisma or vitality, or even my sense of humor about sex. Finally, last year, I went to see another plastic surgeon—this was the third. He said yes, he could do a reconstruction and that it was really easier doing it on both sides because he can match the inserts and not worry about trying to balance the implant with the natural breast.

I was in the hospital for five days. There was very little pain, just a trifle of discomfort afterwards. It's fantastic how quickly it happens. I'd been one-sided for nine years, no-sided for four years. And then, presto, I had a bosom again. Not as large as the original one. No more Marilyn Monroe for me. It's smaller, more delicate—maybe Grace Kelly, the understated, ladylike look.

Anyway, it's wonderful. But I do have a problem. You can't let me loose in a lingerie department because I buy everything in sight. I can't resist all the filmy, beautiful underwear. I have gossamer bras in every color you can imagine. Now I can wear wispy styles, all lace or just a bit of sheer fabric and lace. I have to make up for all the time lost, and for the uncomfortable substitutes I had used in the past.

The most wonderful thing is that I've found my voice again. I didn't sing after the second mastectomy. I couldn't. That was a great loss to me because singing had been an important part of my life.

Now my voice is back, it's as if I'm reborn. The breasts feel soft and natural. The scars are barely visible. I'd say my reconstruction is a complete success. In fact, I'm crazy about it.

5

Now, What about the Other Breast?

After the reconstruction, people were very careful with me, just as they are after you've had a cancer experience. When they meet you on the street after cancer surgery they say, "Hi, how are you?" and they look right into your eyes, as if they were asking, "How are you *really?* Tell me the *real* truth." They don't know what to do with you. It's a combination of fear and self-consciousness.

So people were cautious. They said little. But I could see them looking at me out of the corner of their eyes. They were sizing me up, studying my silhouette. Which one was it?

One man actually asked the question, "Which one is the new one?" I was offended by him. I thought the question was unnecessary.

Now, looking back, I wonder what I did expect. I found people's hesitancy disconcerting. But when a question was asked, it was just as disturbing. Maybe there isn't any proper etiquette for a situation like this. I think mostly my friends were worried that I'd done a wrong thing, that I'd done something that was going to make me terribly sick all over again. I had a feeling they were carrying on private conversations like "Why couldn't we talk her out of this madness?" "Yes, we really shouldn't have let her take this risk." Some friends had cornered Jules earlier and suggested he persuade me to let well enough alone.

But I'd come this far, and now I was going to walk the rest of the way. That meant another operation to reduce my natural breast and construct an areola on the new one. I alternately embraced and fought this idea. One day I'd be annoyed that I had to stuff a piece of foam into my bra over the implant to make it symmetrical with the other side. At that point I'd be sure that I wanted my right breast reduced. Then it would strike me that the surgeon would be cutting into my one good breast and throwing away part of it. What if it didn't work out right? What if something went wrong? Maybe I should quit at this point, not tempt fate, not take this step into the unknown.

I wrestled with the dilemma day and night. Should I? Shouldn't I? It was hard to resolve. Even though I had a new breast, I was still involved with a contrivance—that bit of foam I had to slip into my bra to fill out the contours and give my new left breast the same cup size as the one on the right. I was nearly back to where I'd been in the beginning—but not all the way. With clothes, I looked fine. But without, I was Picasso's unbalanced lady. To be really easy with myself, to get *all* the way back to where I'd been, I knew I had to take the next step.

The hardest part of reaching a decision was not having anyone to talk to. Earlier there had been no one with whom I could share my thoughts and feelings about the reconstruction. And now, again, I felt totally isolated. No other woman I knew had ever wrestled with the decision of whether or not to have her remaining good breast operated on to match her newly rebuilt one. There was no organization to turn to for counseling.

(Reach to Recovery, an organization founded in 1952 by Terese Lasser who had undergone a mastectomy herself, was doing a fine job of giving peer support to breast cancer patients. Today Mrs. Lasser sees a very promising future for breast reconstruction and views it as an important step forward. But at the time I'm talking about, her group had no advice to offer on reconstruction. As for cutting down the other breast to

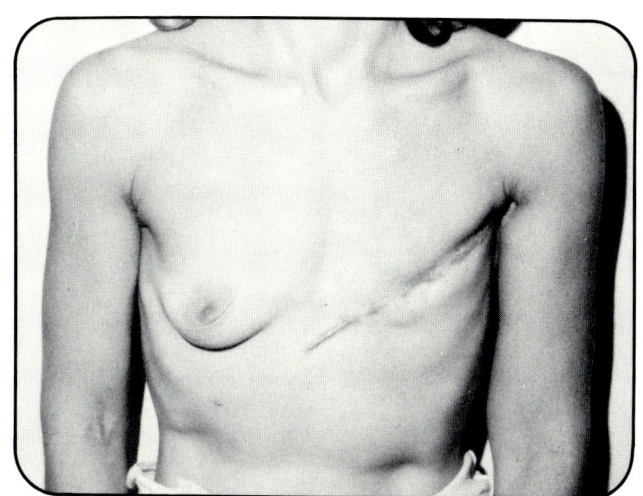

Dr. Randolph Guthrie—Left Modified Radical Mastectomy

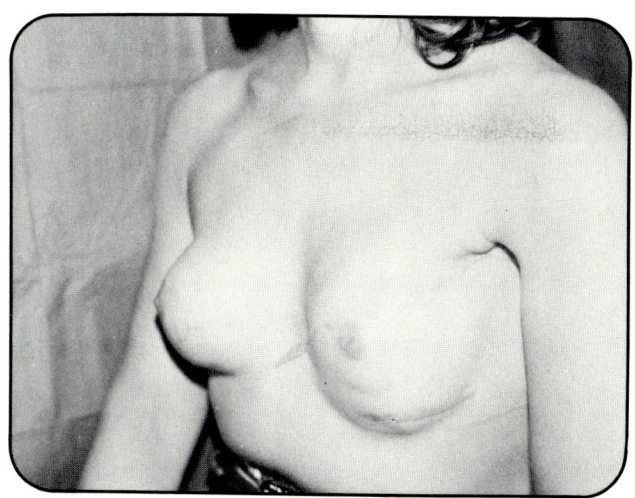

With Silicon Gel Implants and Augmentation of Natural Breast

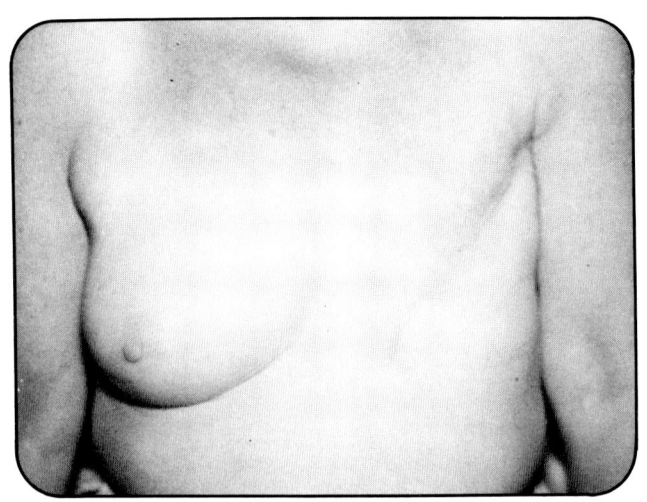
Dr. Saul Hoffman—Modified Radical Mastectomy

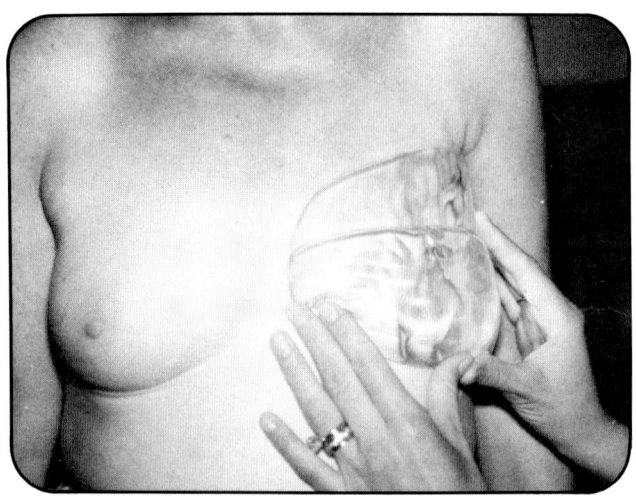
Wax Impression for Moulage for Flat Breast Contour

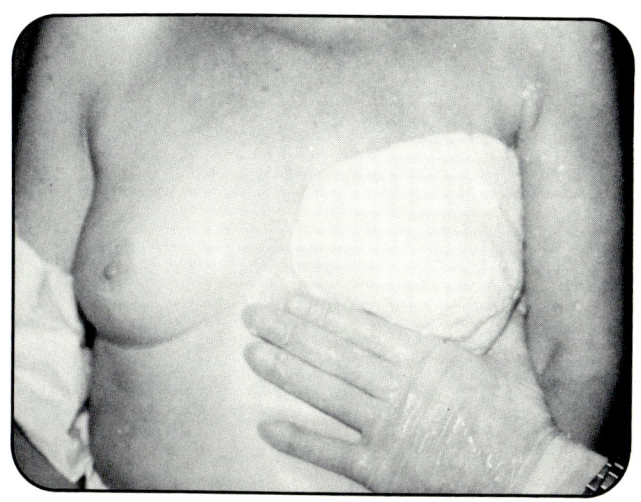
Custom-Designed Prosthesis Held in Place

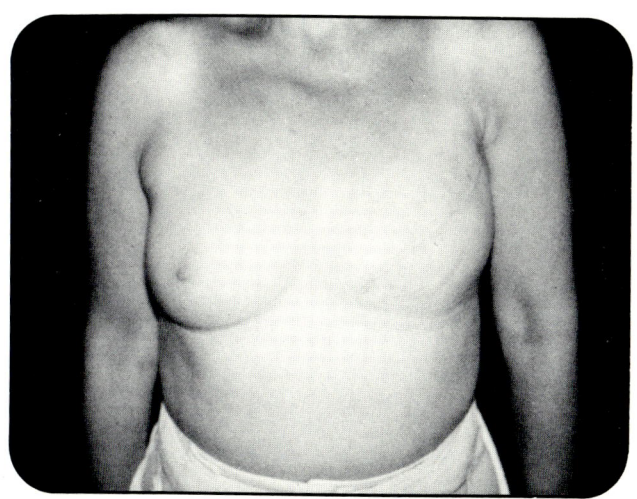
Breast Reconstructed without Areola

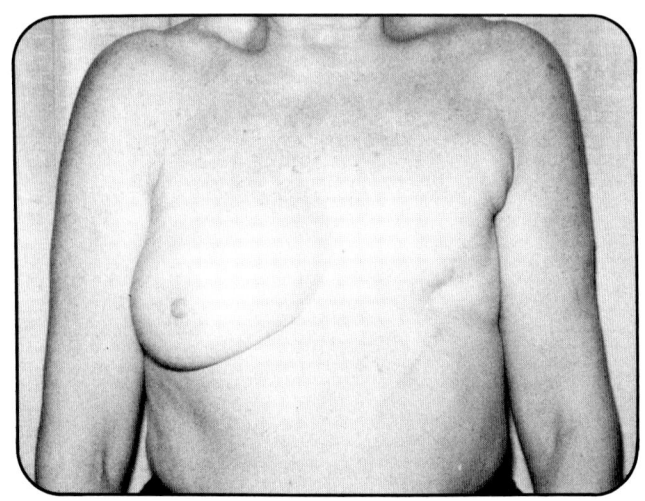

Dr. Saul Hoffman—Modified Radical Mastectomy

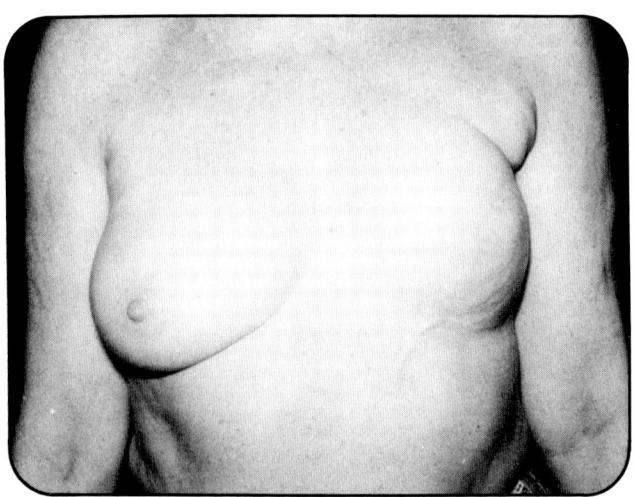

Reconstructed with Saline-Filled Prosthesis

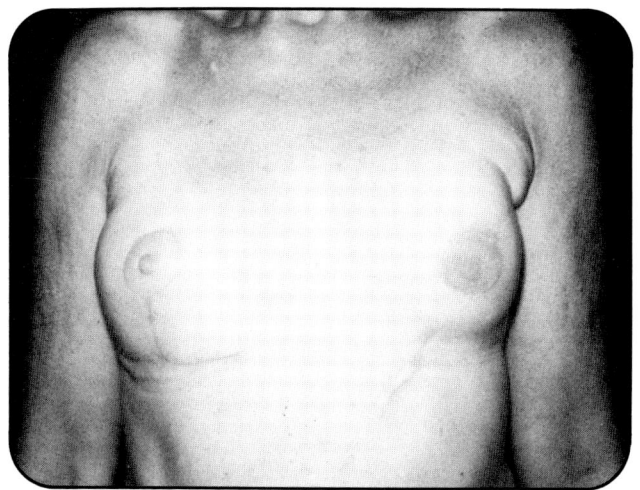

Graft from Labia to Create Nipple and Reduction of Natural Breast

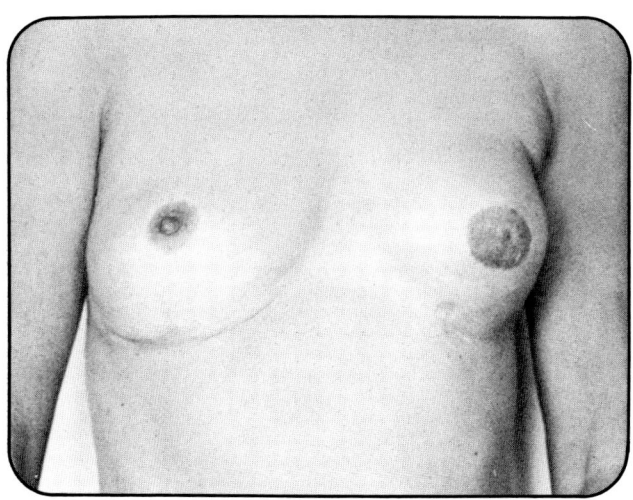

Several Years after Reconstruction

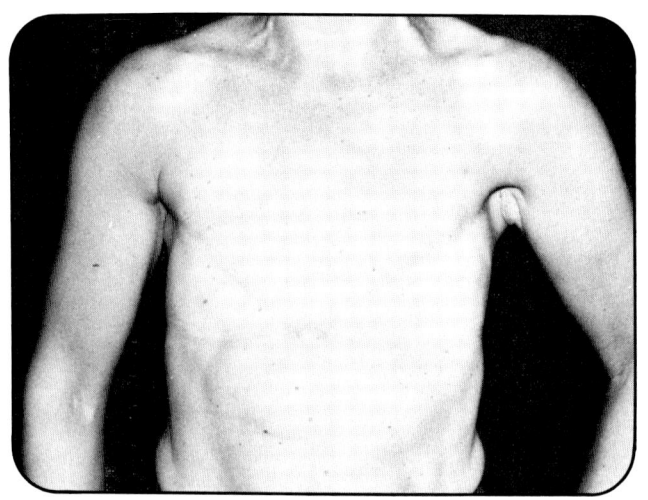

Dr. Saul Hoffman—Bilateral Mastectomy

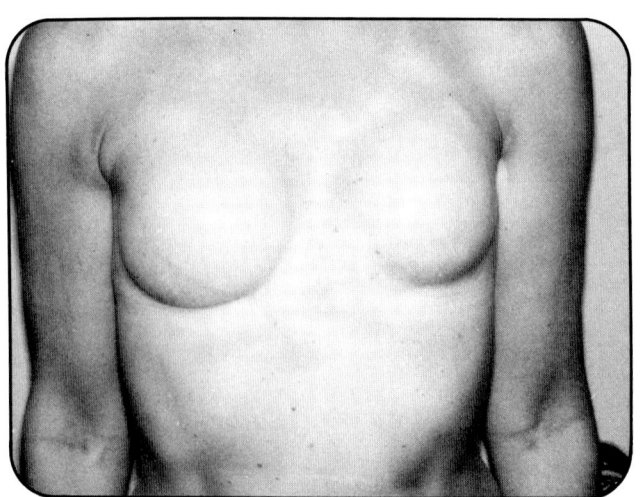

Reconstructed with Saline-filled Prosthesis

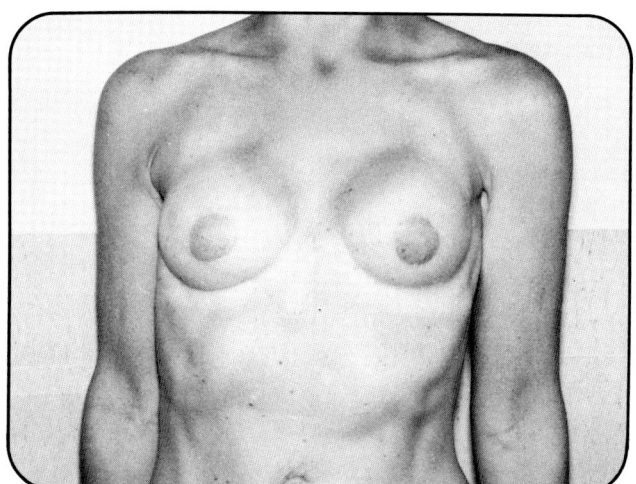

With Areola Grafted from Labia

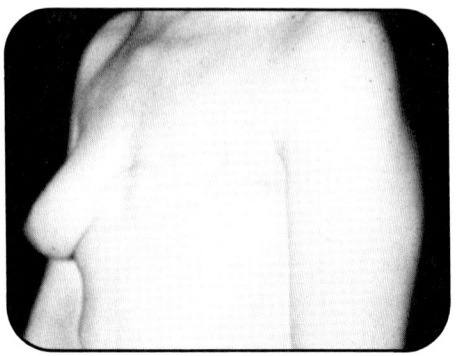

Dr. Saul Hoffman—Left Modified Mastectomy with Transverse Incision

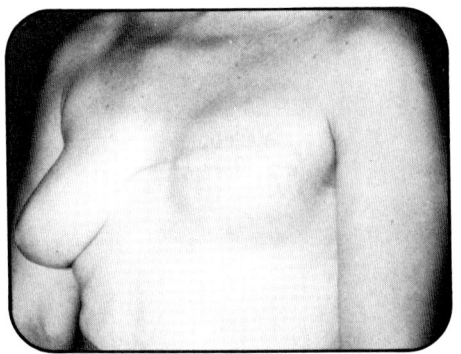

Reconstructed Implant Several Months Later

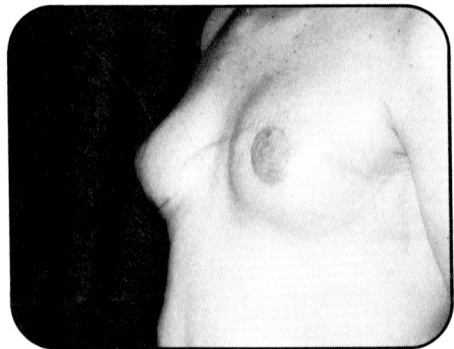

Natural Breast Reduced, with Simulated Areola over Implant

match—that seemed too far-out a notion for serious people to contemplate or discuss.)

My husband could not share in the tension and turmoil I felt as I struggled with the decision about reshaping my good breast. My mother's greatest concern was that I keep secret the fact that I'd had cancer. Of course, I disagreed with her. "It's nothing to be ashamed of," I told her. "It isn't as if I'd had a venereal disease." But she still had so many fears about my health and about cancer itself that I knew it was impossible to talk to her about the new surgery I was considering.

The only one I could talk to was my doctor. Fortunately for me, Dr. Hoffman had a very positive attitude. He firmly urged me to go ahead with the reduction. He knew that in addition to my fears about cutting into the good breast, I was terribly troubled by the question of continued sensitivity in the nipple of the breast after it was reduced. The nipple would have to be snipped off and sewed back on higher up on the curve of the breast. You can imagine how much that idea disturbed me. Dr. Hoffman assured me that the nipple usually continues to have sensitivity in its new position. But I had my doubts. I had doubts about the whole procedure.

While I spun the decision round and round in my head, the doctor drew diagrams on my chest during my visits to his office. He drew a small circle on the implanted breast to indicate where the nipple would be located. Then I'd raise my arm and he'd say, "No, with your arm up, I think it has to go here," and he'd erase his mark and reposition it.

Because my reduced breast would not maintain the exact contour achieved at the time of reduction and would drop a bit as time passed, it would have to be shaped in a way that would make the nipple a trifle high at the beginning. Then as time and gravity did their work, the nipples would eventually come out even. This was something else to worry about.

I really had a high quota of worries.

Should I put myself through another hospital stay and another bout with general anesthesia?

Should I risk having a surgeon, even my trusted Dr. Hoffman, cut into the tissues of the only breast I had left?

Should I take a chance that this nipple, again the only one I had left, would lose its sensitivity?

Suppose something went wrong and the rebuilt breast and the reduced one did not match? Then I would have gone through all this trouble for nothing.

Eventually, of course, I made up my mind to go ahead. My goal was wholeness and symmetry, and this was the only way to achieve it. But I am sure you will believe me when I tell you that even after I checked into the hospital for the new surgery, I was so terrified of the operating room that I found myself tempted to repack my bag and run. Jean, you can still pin a note on the pillow and go home, a timid voice inside my head whispered. I tuned it out.

Conversation

ELISE

Elise, an attractive woman of forty-eight, has been twice married and divorced. She has no children. She is still making up her mind about reconstruction.

Elise, what was your first reaction to mastectomy?
Hysteria. When my doctor told me what was wrong, I thought I was dying of cancer. I thought it would be a slow, painful death. And I thought I wanted to go out fast, rather than suffer. My doctor presented my situation to me as very grave. He thought it was a bad case.

You have a man friend. What was his reaction?
We've been living together for ten years. He has a wife who will not divorce him. He loves me and is totally devoted to me. After the mastectomy his reaction was that I was alive and nothing else mattered. That made me very angry, because once I grasped the fact that I had lost a breast, I forgot all about dying and decided the absolute worst had already happened to me. He thought the fact that I lived was enough to be grateful for. But I didn't see it that way. I didn't see much of anything to be grateful for.

That's interesting, because that was my reaction too. Losing the breast was the most important thing. The cancer was kind of remote and unreal.
Well, I understood the cancer. I knew I was cancerous and that meant from here on in I was in trouble. I'd lost a sister-in-law from it and I knew how bad it can be.

How long was it before you pulled yourself together?
I think the period before was worse than the period after. I had to wait three weeks to get into the hospital. The first week it didn't quite set in my head that I had cancer and had to have a breast removed, so for one week I was rather calm. I even gave two dinner parties. At the end of the week, the surgeon told me that he would probably have to do a radical and I would probably have to have chemotherapy twice a week. The next two weeks, while I was waiting for a hospital bed, I absolutely went bananas. I drank and smoked every night until I could fall asleep. I cried every single night for two weeks. My guy listened and put up with it. He didn't know what to do with me.

In the hospital they were supposed to take me at ten oclock. At eleven-thirty they still hadn't taken me. I asked, "What's going on?" The nurse said, "Well, they usually take the easy case first." Obviously the easy case didn't turn out to be an easy case. The doctor had told me that if I was an easy case it would be forty-five minutes, and if a difficult case three and a half hours. Difficult meant radical surgery.

I was still in my room at twelve o'clock. Then they took me from my room and put me in a hallway where all the doctors were dialing their girlfriends for dates. The nurse was undressing me with people walking by. They didn't knock me out because they didn't know when the surgeon would be ready. I got into the operating room and looked up at the clock—it was ten after one. It was after six when I woke up in the recovery room. So I knew then that I had lost my breast.

When I got to my room, my boyfriend said, "It was a success, you're alive." Well, I didn't really expect to die on the table, so I was very angry with him. Very angry. The ten-day period in the hospital with people and flowers and gifts, you sort of get lost. You're in the hands of people who are taking very good care of you. That helps pull you through. Then you go home and you're alone during the day. Soon you tell friends you're busy or you're tired, but you're not. You just don't want to be bothered with anybody. Then you go back to work.

What was the reaction of your friends?
Totally sympathetic. But there's always somebody who says the wrong thing. There was a woman who kept calling up and saying, "You're behaving like a child. It's nothing." My doctor had already told me I was a disaster case. I think the proper phone call is one in which the caller wishes you good luck or says "I'm very sorry it's happened." If you can't find the right words, just say good-bye and hang up. Calling up and saying, "What's a breast?" doesn't help the person who's lost one.

But I understand that your nodes were negative, so you weren't a disaster case after all.
That's right. But what *really* kept it from being a disaster was that my boyfriend was with me constantly.

How did it affect you sexually?
I used to run around naked. I don't do that any more. But otherwise sexually, there isn't any change.

No changes at all?
Well, I guess I have to admit that my degree of interest in sex is not the same as when I had two breasts. It would be a lie to say it's the same. Especially if you've had a good figure all your life as I had, and your breasts have been a primary factor and if you've run around in a bikini for twenty years, then it's like a new world and not a very good world when suddenly you're all covered up.

How did you learn about reconstruction?
The day of my operation was the day of the article in the *Times* and your picture in the paper. My office cut it out and brought it to me the next day.

Two weeks before the operation *Harper's Bazaar* ran nine articles about cancer written by various people. It was very informative—especially if you were involved. I read them all very thoroughly. So I knew something about reconstruction. I have a friend who is vain and involved with appearance, and she had said to me, "Have your nipple banked." I asked my surgeon's secretary about that. She said he'd done it only once —for a patient who'd refused to have the cancer removed unless he saved the nipple. He didn't want to, but he did it for her.

I told her about the articles in *Harper's Bazaar*. She said I shouldn't take those women's magazines too seriously. "But some of the articles are written by doctors," I told her, "so it's not as if it's some gossip in a trashy newspaper."

I guess I was in too much of a fog to pursue it. Now I think if I had to do it over, I would pursue it more. I think my surgeon should have said to me, "You know you can have your nipple banked. I don't do that sort of operation, but so-and-so does." I was not given the alternatives that I should have known about. I never had a choice. I was not given the right to make this important decision about myself. I think the doctor owes it to the patient to give her all the information available.

Did you discuss reconstruction with your boyfriend?

Yes, and he's been for it from the beginning, but he isn't pushing me because he doesn't want to be blamed if it doesn't come out right. He wants me to do it for me. Everybody thinks I should do it. I'm the only one who is wavering.

Why, what's your problem?

Wait until you hear what I've been through. I've seen three different plastic surgeons and gotten three different opinions. Doctor Number One in New York wants $2,500 for the job and he'll use a silicone implant that is filled with a saline solution and he makes a vertical incision in the side. He explained to me very carefully why he thinks that's the best procedure.

Dr. Number Two, also in New York, says he'll make the opening under the breast and he'll use a rough-textured implant that is made to order according to my measurements. His fee is $4,000. And he told me what good results he gets with his procedure.

Dr. Number Three is on the West Coast—yes, I went out to California to see him because several friends have told me what marvelous work he does. Well, he wants $5,000 and he uses a saline-filled implant and makes a horizontal incision. He takes a piece of the remaining nipple to make a nipple for the new breast. Then he tells me there's a chance I may lose sensation in the good nipple when he divides it. Well, that gets me really scared. After that, he goes on to say that I have a 20 percent chance of getting cancer in the other breast, and it might be a good idea to do a prophylactic mastectomy on the good breast to forestall a future cancer. That scares me even more.

What about reducing the good breast in size—did anyone mention that?

Oh yes, that's another thing. Both New York surgeons pointed out that my good breast hangs but the reconstruction doesn't. So they want to operate on the good one.

To add to everything else, I saw some reconstructions on TV recently, and I can't say they filled me with confidence. They showed one breast high, one low, the nipple too far to the right or too far to the left. The results weren't at all like what you have. Your reconstruction looks really natural. But those things on television certainly didn't.

So where do you stand now?

Right now, I'm in a to-hell-with-it stage. I think I'll take a breather. I'm going to mull over all the possibilities and take my time before I make up my mind. I think I'll eventually decide in favor of reconstruction because I don't like being disfigured. But I'm going to wait a little until the confusion settles.

6

Whole, at Last

Again I was wheeled up to the operating room and given full anesthesia. When I awoke, it was incredible. I remember lying in bed and seeing two heaving things on my chest that looked absolutely beautiful to me.

On the left side there was just a bit of bandage over the reddish circle called the areola that had been transplanted from the outer lip of the labia tissue near the vagina. I learned later that what surgeons do to create an areola by this technique is to cut away a very thin circle—thinner than tissue paper—of the pinkish tissue from the labial area. A circle of equal size at the designated place on the breast is prepared by a method that is very much like skin peeling and is done with a high-speed abrading tool. The labial transplant is then placed on the exposed underskin of the breast and stitched in place with the tiniest embroidery stitches you can imagine.

Perhaps this is the point to tell you, if you don't already know, that today's skilled plastic surgeon operates with a delicacy and precision that is absolutely unbelievable to the ordinary lay person. I've seen the faces of children, born with terrible congenital deformities, that have been rebuilt, step by step, in twenty or more surgical procedures. And when this work is done by a truly gifted plastic surgeon, the scars are such feathery tracings they are hardly visible to the naked eye. Plastic surgeons can create missing lips or eyelids out of bits and pieces of tissue from other parts of the body, and do it so beautifully that the casual observer never guesses what has taken place.

To surgeons of this caliber, a breast and nipple rebuilding, such as I had, is one of the easier procedures on their daily operating schedule. Their magic hands have devised some astonishing ways to create a nipple—which we will discuss in a later chapter.

My right side was more heavily bandaged than my left, but even so, I could see the top of the breast and the lovely matching curves on both sides. Where, before the latest surgery, one side had been high and the other low, now both were high, rounded and very youthful-looking. And there between the breasts was that most delicious of things—cleavage. It's funny how something that most of us take for granted becomes precious when it no longer exists. I, of course, had lost cleavage completely with the mastectomy and it had not really been returned with the first stage of reconstruction because the breasts were at different levels. But now here it was in full flower—a joy to have.

It was May, a time of renewal, and I had never before been so aware of the symbolism of the season. When the bandages came off, I had a triumphant feeling of having conquered the hurts and losses of the past, of having erased the whole cancer experience.

Now I really was back where I had started, both in my physical state and in my self-image. It wasn't that I had suddenly achieved youthfulness and sexiness. It was simply that I was back where I had been. I went into a high such as I had never known before. I was absolutely elated.

Once again I could wear two-piece bathing suits—even bikinis. That may not seem like much to you, especially if you don't like bikinis, but it was important for me. It was important because it made me feel like everybody else. I could watch television in my nightgown without worrying every time the doorbell rang. I could play tennis and then go to the locker room without the fear that someone would discover how I looked. I even began to go around braless in public—something I had never done in my life. It was exhilarating. At home I could walk about nude once again—no more need to hide that absent part of my body.

In fact, my joy was almost more than I could handle. I wanted to show everyone. To my amazement, most people weren't especially enthusiastic about being shown. In fact, my friends were quite squeamish. Nobody actually asked to look. And when I insisted on displaying the surgeon's splendid handiwork to my women friends, most took a quick, almost furtive glance and turned away.

The only ones who looked carefully—who looked and looked —were those who had already undergone mastectomy. They pelted me with questions. They poked and touched. They could hardly believe their eyes. When I think back I realize that what they looked at at that early stage was really not so gorgeous.

My new breasts were very firm and high. The right one, my own which had been reduced in size and raised, had a prominent horizontal scar along the chest under the curve and a vertical scar from the ribs up to the nipple. The line of stitching around the areola where it had been sewed on was also slightly visible. The left breast showed the old mastectomy scar, now grown considerably fainter with the years, in a long diagonal line from the underarm to the rib area under the breast and continuing for several inches down toward the abdomen. There were stitch marks around the new areola, which was darker than the natural areola on the other side. There was no projecting nipple on that side, only the reddish circle of the areola. And there was an angry-looking vertical scar at the underarm side of the left breast.

All the scars are faded now and some hardly noticeable. But those women who had lost a breast of their own hardly saw the then red, raw scars at all. They saw the symmetry and the completeness. They saw my happiness. And as they contrasted their own amputation with my wholeness, their own constant reminder of cancer in their bodies with my erasure of that reminder, I could see the idea taking shape in their heads. They were putting themselves in my place. And they were thinking that maybe they, too, could be whole again.

Less than a week after I was out of the hospital, I was walking down the street when some construction workers whistled at me. My consciousness is sufficiently raised for me to recognize the whistle as an unwelcome attention. But this time I was delighted. I felt like smiling at the whistlers and thanking them, although I wasn't sure I should take the credit myself or pass it on to Dr. Hoffman, whose lovely workmanship had provoked the admiration.

In June I was invited to my first social event, a garden party. Without the prosthesis I felt free and unburdened. I wore a pearl-gray one-piece jumper that was cut very low and had thin spaghetti straps. I had a wonderful feeling of having been restored to where I had been prior to the cancer surgery.

And then I knew what I had to do.

I had to tell women about breast reconstruction. I had to share my discovery.

Conversation

MONICA

Monica is a writer who lives in New York.

Monica, I understand you had your mastectomy in 1974. What was your first reaction?
I guess it was the pleasure of being alive. That's what I felt first. There was no infiltration of the lymph nodes, so that made me feel even better. The relief of having it over with and being all right blotted out everything else.

When did you first hear about reconstruction?
I think I first learned about it from a magazine article, but it wasn't a very positive introduction. It showed some cases from South America and they looked so grotesque to me that I was really turned off. But then more recently, as you know, I heard about it through you. An editor working on your book told me about you, we met, I was impressed with what had happened to you and I made an appointment with a plastic surgeon. Now I'm on my way.

How did your family feel about the idea?
You know, that's been one of my problems. I'm not married. Everything I've read since my mastectomy about breast problems—articles in magazines, books by women—talks about it as a family problem. But that wasn't the case with me. My friends were marvelous—very supportive of me. But I guess I had been repressing psychologically a lot of my feelings. I realized my friends who had been so wonderful never broached the problem. My friends were holding back on me because I was holding back on myself.

Has that changed?
Yes, it has, because the prospect of reconstruction has opened it all up for me, and for everybody. I've been talking freely about the reconstruction and once I started talking, my friends did, too, and there's been this wonderful sharing and growing closer.
I also realized how much I had not allowed myself to feel. The prospect of reconstruction forced me to face the fact that I'd been unhappy about myself, about the way I looked, about my incompleteness.
As I made plans for the reconstruction I felt for the first time in a long time that I was in control again. I was not at the dictate—you could even say the mercy—of doctors' decisions. You know, the doctor says, "You *have* to have this biopsy." Then he says, "You *have* to have this breast off." You go along, because you *have* to. But now, with the reconstruction, this time I say what *I* want. It's a wonderful feeling—very healthy, very liberating.

Where are you with reconstruction now?
I've already had some minor preliminaries taken care of. The plastic surgeon had to correct a few small things first. That's done, and now I'm scheduled to have the implant put in in about a month. I had a modified radical, so I'm told the reconstruction will be simple to perform. In my head it's almost as if it's already been done. I'm thinking about buying new clothes. I can see that my future dealings with men will be quite different. I'm looking forward to the whole social scene. I already have a new sense of self. I can't tell you how grateful I am for the idea of reconstruction. It's really changed my life.

7

Going Public

The half a million women now alive who have had breast surgery were the ones I particularly wanted to tell about breast reconstruction. I wanted the message to reach beyond them, to *all* women. With one out of thirteen women now stricken with this dread disease, every woman sooner or later faces in her own life or in the life of a loved relative or friend the specter of breast cancer. All of them, I felt, should know that mutilation is not necessarily final. For those who wish it and for those whose physical condition makes it possible, there is now the option of restoration.

Although I am not a writer and had never attempted anything literary, I decided I'd write an article for one of the women's magazines. That way I could spread the word about breast reconstruction.

I called and wrote letters to several magazines. The editors turned me down. The idea was too new, too uncertain. They weren't interested.

Then a young woman writer got in touch with me after she'd seen some before-and-after photographs of me at a plastic surgery convention. When she asked Dr. Hoffman if she could interview me, he had cleared it with me and I arranged to see her. When we met, I told her how I had tried unsuccessfully to interest several women's magazines in my story and I gave her my material. Later she collaborated with another writer and eventually the story was told in the September 1975 issue of *Good Housekeeping* magazine.

Soon after the *Good Housekeeping* article appeared, I saw on *A.M. New York*, a TV news program, a brief preview of a roundup on plastic surgery which was scheduled for the following day. I went right to the phone, called the station and said, "I heard your announcement about tomorrow's program and I want to tell you that I've had a kind of plastic surgery you may not know about—a breast reconstruction." They told me to get over to the station at once.

I took a cab downtown, went in to see the people in the *A.M. New York* office and showed them my photographs— premastectomy, postmastectomy, first stage of reconstruction and after complete reconstruction. They passed around the photographs, looked at me with stares that bored right through my clothes and they were all saying, "This is marvelous, absolutely marvelous. We never heard of it; we have to do it."

But they were hesitant about showing the pictures on the air. "We have a mixed audience," one of the producers explained to me. "It's a mixed family audience, not just an adult audience."

I was insistent. If they were to interview me, they'd have to show the photographs. I don't know what made me so bold. But I felt this TV show, even though it was seen only in New York, would be a milestone in reaching the public, and I knew the best way to convey the message of reconstruction surgery was to show the pictures. We argued back and forth for quite a while. Eventually they did it my way and the interview went very well. The M.C.s—there were two, a man and a woman —asked me about my mastectomy, my feelings about myself afterwards, my decision to have the breast rebuilt and the results of the plastic surgery.

I answered as simply and matter-of-factly as I could. When the slides were flashed on the screen, I described each one. Lacking then the assurance I now have in talking about myself, I made the commentary impersonal, saying, "Here is a woman after mastectomy." I could not bring myself to say, "This is the way I looked." I went through the series of pictures, talking about a woman, any woman, although, of course, the viewers knew from the interview that *I* had undergone the operations.

As far as I know, this was the first time that breast reconstruction was ever discussed and shown on television. Even though the program did not have a studio audience, there was a strong reaction in the studio afterwards among the staff people and the technicians. The women, especially, crowded around me and asked many questions. One young woman shook my hand and said, "Gee, you've got a lot of courage." Several expressed their relief at knowing that reconstruction existed—in case breast cancer should hit them at some future time. "Now I think I could face it without going crazy," one young woman said. Several asked such pointed questions that I knew they must be thinking of a friend or family member who had undergone cancer surgery.

Later the producer reported back to me that the station had received many calls from viewers congratulating it on doing the program. A few letters were forwarded to me which said things like, "Thank you for doing that. It was very important. We never knew about this."

Most significant, the sky did not fall because a few photographs of bare breasts were shown on a television program that documented the plastic-surgery response to the ravages of breast cancer.

A few months later my husband and I had just returned to New York from a trip to Greece. As I ran to catch a Madison Avenue bus I caught my foot in a manhole. ("Please, a personhole," corrected the doctor who put the cast on my cracked ankle. Obviously someone had been at work on his consciousness.) While the ankle was still keeping me partially homebound I got a phone call from the producers of *Eyewitness News* on ABC–TV. They were doing a program on plastic surgery and had heard about me from *A.M. New York*. Could they interview me? I explained that I had a cast on my leg, but if they wanted to come to my apartment, fine.

The next morning four men arrived with cameras, cables,

lights, equipment. They deployed their stuff around the apartment, sat me in a chair and the interviewer, a very young man, started asking questions. I really had to make an effort not to laugh because he was treating me with such exaggerated deference I knew he thought I was older than Whistler's mother by at least a decade and too fragile to last out the day. He also seemed embarrassed at discussing a topic as indelicate as a woman's breasts. The film they took was terribly overexposed, so I guess the cameraman was just as nervous as the interviewer.

The brief segment about me appeared on the air as part of a program that was chiefly devoted to breast augmentation and reduction. But that didn't matter, because once more the word was going out to women. And that's what I really wanted.

I even became something of an exhibitionist in my cause. At a dinner party one night my hostess introduced me to another guest and said, "I know you two have both had mastectomies, but Jean has gone a step beyond. Gladys, you may want to talk to her about it."

Gladys listened eagerly to the account of my reconstruction. "Would you let me see it?" she asked.

"Sure, let's go to the bathroom." I'd had two martinis and was feeling free and relaxed.

I lowered the shoulder straps of the dress I was wearing. Her eyes opened very wide as she examined me with care. "Do you mind if I show Leonard?" she asked.

Those two martinis were still working. "Not at all," I said.

Leonard crowded into the bathroom with us and gravely scrutinized my bosom. I felt no embarrassment, only a great sense of closeness to Gladys and a feeling of the importance of the moment for her.

Later Jules wasn't all that enthusiastic about my performance. "Do you really have to go that far?" he asked. "Oh, it's just the mechanics of the thing that's so interesting," I told him. "I think Gladys is really going to look into reconstruction." He made no further objections.

Shortly after that, I was asked to make a video tape for the Department of Psychiatry at Beth Israel Hospital. On the tape

I told of my mastectomy, described my desolate feelings afterwards and then discussed the sense of totality gained after reconstruction. I also spoke of the choice of a two-stage mastectomy procedure. The video tape was first used as a teaching film for the staff of the Department of Psychiatry.

Later I was happy to hear the film was being shown to mastectomy patients while they were still in the hospital. I thought of the great value to these women of looking at a film of someone who had had her lost breast rebuilt and who told her story of reconstruction simply and directly. What I wouldn't have given to have seen such a film when I was at the lowest depth of my anguish!

That same year, I was invited to a Breast Cancer Conference at Beth Israel which was attended by dozens of the hospital's physicians, surgeons, interns, residents, nurses and medical students. There was a discussion during which I described my search for reconstruction and my happiness with the result.

The doctors in the audience showed varying degrees of interest. A few asked searching questions. One asked me, "Which hit you first, the fact of cancer or the fact of losing your breast?"

"I was first hit by the loss of my breast. The fact of having cancer only hit me some time later," I told him. It was clear from their comments that for many of the physicians the whole idea of breast reconstruction by plastic surgery was new and challenging. I began to feel that the message was beginning to get across to where it was really needed. High time, too.

Then, toward the end of 1976 the real breakthrough came. I got a phone call from Dee Wedemeyer, a reporter with *The New York Times*, who was doing an article on breast reconstruction. A careful reporter, she did a great deal of research on the subject and interviewed cancer specialists and plastic surgeons in New York, Massachusetts, Texas, New Jersey, Florida, Pennsylvania. The extensive article she wrote appeared in the *Times* on December 9, 1976, under the headline "After Mastectomy: The Options for Breast Reconstruction."

It included an interview with me and was illustrated with my photograph.

In the text, Dee Wedemeyer mentioned a questionnaire sent by Vanderbilt University in 1975 to 1,536 plastic surgeons in the United States and Canada. Of the 795 who replied, 359 said they had performed 1,186 breast reconstructions. That figure astonished me. I had no idea the practice had become that widespread—and in so short a time.

The article pointed out the psychological advantages of reconstruction and quoted Dr. Robert M. Goldwyn, associate clinical professor of surgery at the Harvard Medical School, as saying, "Remember, this is a group of women who knew what they looked like before and have generally a reminder (the remaining breast) of what they looked like before. Reconstruction helps them to get on with living a normal life without having to worry about it."

Dr. Thomas D. Cronin, clinical professor of plastic surgery at the Baylor College of Medicine in Texas, a pioneer in the development of the silicone gel implant, which was used originally to enlarge undersized breasts and later adapted for reconstruction, estimated that as many as 80 percent of the women who had undergone mastectomies could have some degree of reconstruction.

Dr. Jerome Urban, attending surgeon at Memorial Sloan-Kettering Cancer Center in New York, one of the country's leading cancer surgeons, said he had no objection to reconstruction provided that the removal of the cancer had priority. "It is better to have a live patient than a reconstructed one," Dr. Urban said. "Otherwise I think more power to the plastic people." Dr. Urban is the surgeon who performed the mastectomies on Happy Rockefeller, the wife of the former Vice President.

Dr. D. Ralph Millard, Jr., professor of plastic surgery at the University of Miami School of Medicine in Florida, described the more complicated reconstructions following radical mastectomies and severe radiation damage. Some of these procedures, he explained, require four hospitalizations and complex operations that in slow stages transfer skin and fatty tissue from the abdominal area to the breast. "If they want it, they can do it," Dr. Millard said.

The only dissenting opinion was expressed by Dr. C. D. Haagensen, emeritus professor of surgery at Columbia University. "Madness," he said of reconstruction. "You mustn't flirt with breast cancer. It is a terrible disease." Dr. Haagensen believed that cancer could be spread by another operation and thought most of the reconstructions he had seen were not aesthetically successful. (Dr. Haagensen's views are discussed further on pp. 105–6.)

After the article appeared, I questioned Dee Wedemeyer about her enormous interest in the subject. She seemed much too young to have had personal involvement in breast cancer, although I knew very well it does sometimes strike women in their twenties. She told me that all women have a strong sense of being threatened by breast cancer, and that she had pursued the subject of reconstruction as intensely as she did because she thought it was one of the most important women's news stories of the year. She was convinced it would affect the lives of thousands of women. I agreed with her completely.

I had never seen so much basic, helpful information on the subject gathered together in one place. I had never before heard so many prominent surgeons speak favorably of reconstruction. In fact, I'd had no idea that so many reconstructions were being done in so many parts of the country. I knew this article would be a turning point, that it would have an immense effect.

The newspaper was hardly on the stands when my telephone began to ring. It rang constantly. Women said to me, "I never heard of this before. I want to know more." Women asked, "How did you learn about reconstruction? How do I find a surgeon?" Women came to see me with their stories of fear and anger.

One conversation among all the others stood out in my mind and convinced me that I was on the right track in wanting to help others. An attractive young woman who had just had a biopsy that indicated a malignancy walked into my apartment in a jersey dress that crossed over in front and emphasized her lovely bosom. Despite her confident carriage, her eyes were glazed with a sick fear. "I know I should let the surgeon operate, but I can't do it. I just can't do it," she said, almost in tears. "I'm not going to let him cut off my breast. I don't want to live that way."

I gave her some tea and calmed her down a little by asking her about her work as a textile designer. Then we got back to her medical problem. Her doctor wanted to perform a mastectomy and insisted that it was urgent to do it quickly because of the location of the lesion and the particular pathology indicated by her biopsy. She had refused. There was no way she would allow him to amputate her breast. She would have the lump removed, at the very most. But maybe she'd skip the whole thing and let nature take its course. In doing that, she knew she might be sentencing herself to an early death.

To try to persuade her to undergo the necessary surgery, her doctor had shown her photographs of reconstructed breasts. But the photographs were poor and the rebuilt breasts looked hard, tight and quite unnatural.

"But you're happy with your reconstruction," she said to me almost accusingly. "How come? The pictures I've seen look so awful."

She asked to see what I looked like. I told her I'd be glad to show her what had been done for me and I did my, by now, customary striptease. She looked at me in amazement. By this time my scars had faded down to faint pink lines. As I have mentioned, the nipples are different from each other, but the contours on both sides are equally rounded, the skin smooth and soft and the breasts feel remarkably alike to the touch.

"My God, you look so much better than the pictures," she gasped. "You look wonderful." Then she let out a long, slow sigh, as if a terrible struggle had come to an end.

"All right, I'll do it. I'll call my doctor today and I'll have the surgery," she said. She was crying hard now, but these tears were different. They were an uprushing of relief, almost of happiness. For now she knew she would live and there was a strong possibility she would live with her body relatively unblemished. She kissed me when she left, as if we were old close friends.

She had the mastectomy that same week and her plastic surgeon was present at the operation. He took the nipple from the removed breast—it was not involved in the malignancy—and banked it by temporarily attaching it to her groin. Some time later her breast was rebuilt, using her own nipple. The redone breast was so close in size and shape to her remaining natural one that no further correction was necessary.

She came to see me again eight months later, wearing that same revealing, cross-over jersey dress. She looked marvelous. Her smile was radiant. She tried to thank me, but I cut her off as gently as I could. I told her, "Don't thank me. Just turn it around and help me reach other women and doctors. You have a terrific story to tell. Go out and tell it."

Conversation

VALERIE

Valerie, the mother of two daughters, had a radical mastectomy fifteen years ago.

I like showing my reconstruction to you because I think it's very encouraging. What do you think?
Yes, it is and I'm amazed that the labial tissue used for the nipple matches so well.

It really does. Sometimes I give myself tests. I went into a sauna not long ago and stripped. I was among a lot of women, strangers to me. We talked, but nobody looked at me. I didn't even get a sidelong glance—the kind you do from a woman who's had a few biopsies and is very alert to any changes in the breast.
I go to the sauna, too. I decided that losing a breast wasn't a punishment. So I went, although it took me years to get up the courage. Nothing much happened. Hardly anyone looked and no one said anything.

That's very courageous of you. I kept myself hidden before I had the reconstruction. I guess I thought it was aesthetically offensive to people.
I felt that way with my daughters. They were very young and I never allowed them to see me. My eighteen-year-old daughter and I went on a long trip together last year. That was before I began the reconstruction. I decided it was time to stop hiding. The funny thing is that she was so modest that I never really saw *her* the whole time.

What made you consider having reconstruction after fifteen years?
A friend of mine did all the research. She went around talking to doctors and was really avid to have it done for herself. I was only mildly interested, but I did say to her, "Let me know what you find out." She went ahead with a doctor in Stamford, Connecticut, and was so overjoyed with the results that she showed me her reconstruction. "Gee, it really looks good," I said. "It's really terrific." And I began to think it might be a good thing for me to do.

I guess I have a particular feeling about life. I once heard a biologist in California say that our natural life span should be three hundred years and we theoretically could live that long if we could wipe out all the things that get in the way. That really intrigued me—the idea that life could go on for a very long time. And then I began to think that since I have only this body, I might as well do the best with it that I can.

I understand you've gone to Germany for your reconstruction. Why is that?
I'd heard of a doctor there who does really remarkable work. I had a radical, so it's quite a job to do me. This doctor uses part of the stomach to make the pectoral muscle.

That must be the procedure using omentum—the fatty tissue in the abdomen.
I guess that's it. Anyway, he prides himself on filling in the whole area and his goal is that it should look better than new. Not just passable. He says I should be able to wear a bikini. And I really like that.

Where are you in the reconstruction now?
The plastic surgeon has completed the first stage. He's moved the tissue from the upper abdomen to fill the hollow and now I'm waiting for it to heal and then I'll have the second stage—the construction of the breast. He did another thing for

me. I've had some cysts that keep popping up in my good breast. They've been aspirated [the fluid drawn out] three times, and before I went to Germany there was some talk about doing a subcutaneous mastectomy. But the doctor in Germany removed the cyst and made a fine-line incision around the nipple. You can hardly see the scar. So I'm delighted with that.

Have you come up against any negative attitudes about your reconstruction?

Only from a doctor who said you couldn't really tell how it would shape up later on. But nobody's mentioned anything about inciting disease.

The big problem seems to be for women to communicate with their doctors to let them know it's not enough to remove the cancer. They want something done about the deformity.

The trouble is that some plastic surgeons tell you it looks like a golf ball. Who wants that? Or they say, "You're over fifty, why are you interested?"

Did you ever get used to looking at yourself without that breast?

I think after a while I just came to accept it. On that trip I mentioned I went to a famous cave in India on a solid rock island. There's a hollowed-out temple to the god Shiva with tremendous columns and huge bas-reliefs depicting episodes in the god's life. In one of them he is half man, half woman. So he has one breast. My daughter looked at it and said, "It reminds me of someone I know."

I remember when I first came home from the hospital after the mastectomy, I was taking a bath and my mother was helping me get out of the tub. She looked at me and burst into tears. I wasn't happy about it—but I wasn't all that upset. They had told me before the biopsy, "It's nothing." I have a close relative who's a surgeon, and he examined me and said, "It's nothing, nothing." When I woke up and saw the big bandage,

I said to the doctor, "It was something, wasn't it?" He said, "Yes, I'm sorry—it was." And he said to me, "Your husband is so upset—you really have to be brave." That stuck in my mind—that I was supposed to be brave because *he* was so upset. It didn't occur to me until years later that *I* had the right to be upset.

8

Women Respond

I began to hear from women in a way I had never imagined. The messages reached me by mail, by telephone, in personal visits. Pathetic letters piled up from women who told of bitter unhappiness after mastectomy, ruined careers, broken marriages, drinking, even suicide attempts. Women rang my doorbell—with or without appointments. They showered me with questions about reconstruction. They poured out their stories of misery and anger. It was truly an odd experience; these women were all total strangers one minute and the very next minute were revealing their innermost thoughts and uncovering their mutilated bodies for me to see.

I've never had a sense of mission about my life, but I couldn't help being aware that in certain ways I was uniquely prepared for these intimate encounters. For the ten years I had worked on the mammography study at HIP, as part of my job I'd interviewed women on an extremely personal level and come to accept cancer as an everyday fact of life. Then I'd had my own cancer experience. That had taught me that dealing factually with other people's cancer and having it yourself are totally different matters. Maybe it's a little like the difference between writing specifications for seat belts and nearly pitching through the windshield in a head-on collision. You have to go through it yourself for the reality to hit home.

At any rate, here I was, in the right place at the right time, listening, learning, sharing, guiding, exploring with these deeply troubled women who had so suddenly come into my life. What did they have to say?

Some of them were women who had no personal problem, but were moved to sympathy and a desire to help others. Many said the relief of knowing there was an alternative to the permanent disfiguring of a mastectomy made the prospect, if it should occur in the future, much less terrifying to them.

Others were women I'd known in earlier periods in my life. They'd seen my name in the newspaper and gotten in touch again because they wanted to assist in some way. For example, the mother of a childhood friend of my son wrote that she was aware of all the suffering and asked if she could address envelopes or do anything that might be useful.

I heard from professional people who wanted more information or had suggestions to offer. A dentist inquired if plastic surgeons had ever thought of using gum tissue to rebuild a nipple. The coordinator of the Mastectomy Advisory Programme in Belfast, Ireland, wrote to tell me that the United States was far ahead of her country and asked for further information.

Then there were the women who had already had reconstruction. Most of them were happy, almost exploding with exuberance, wanting to tell me their stories and hear more about mine. Several suggested that we band together in some way to spread the word about reconstruction.

From Illinois a woman wrote: "I had a mastectomy twenty years ago and a reconstruction just last year. I am so happy with it I would be eager to help others if I could. Please let me know how."

There were some women who had had reconstructions that were not satisfactory for one reason or another. One woman who came to see me had been operated on several years earlier, and her implant, a type no longer in use, had shrunk and hardened. (I quietly blessed my good surgeon for not letting me plunge impetuously into reconstruction before the devices and techniques had been perfected.) Once this woman saw what

I looked like, she made an appointment with a new doctor to have her implant replaced.

A widow who had had a radical mastectomy showed me a restoration that had not worked. Her plastic surgeon had tried to fill the cavity left by the removed pectoral muscle with a special prosthesis, but it had not remained in place. Now she still had the cavity near her armpit and a protrusion in the wrong place near her collarbone. What could I tell her, except perhaps to see another doctor?

I realized, when I spoke to this woman, what a cautious line I had to tread in my conversations and correspondence. I could not offer medical advice or even express a medical opinion. Women would have to see their own doctor or a different doctor when it came to any aspect of their disease or the technical side of reconstruction. I could only open their eyes to the options and the possibilities. I could show them what had been done for me. From there on they would have to take their own steps.

The most pressured women who consulted me were those who did not yet have cancer for sure but were faced with the imminent possibility. I talked to four of these women in a two-week period—two who were afraid to go for mammography and two who were too terrified of losing a breast to face a biopsy. Each time, when I saw the relief flooding over them after they looked at me, I was struck with the urgency of spreading the word about reconstruction not only as an aesthetic solution to an ugly problem but also as a method of saving lives—often young lives full of promise.

Mrs. L., still in her thirties, the mother of four, had had cysts and benign breast problems for some time. Now her doctor wanted her to have a mammogram. She was so convinced the diagnosis would be cancer that she had been afraid to make the appointment. But if she saw what a rebuilt breast looked like . . . perhaps then she could get up her courage.

For months Mrs. S. had refused to have a mastectomy. She had decided she would rather die than live with her body mutilated. But when she read the article in the *Times*, she went right to her doctor and consented to the surgery. With knowledge of reconstruction, she was willing to take the step necessary to save her life. Now she wanted to thank me.

Finally there were the women, the great majority of my callers, who had parted with a breast, either recently or even decades earlier, and who echoed the same refrain: "Tell me, tell me, I never heard of this before."

A woman wrote from Virginia: "I feel very much as you did —that there has to be another way, beyond stuffing something into your bra. Now I am looking for a plastic surgeon to see what he can do for me. You deserve a bouquet for reminding us that the physical has to be rebuilt to overcome the psychological damage."

Here is a particularly sensitive letter from a woman in Connecticut:

> I hope you will not think it presumptuous of me to write to you, but every day that has gone by since I read of your reconstructive surgery has been one of turmoil and indecision.
>
> As you have probably gathered, I had a radical mastectomy three years ago, and ever since have been haunted by the inescapable reminder of "disease" as well as disfigurement. I also continue to be slightly upset by not having been informed, or of informing myself, for that matter, of the options available for implants and reconstruction. I suppose, like everyone else at first, the relief of being alive was enough.
>
> The medical response to my timid request for a possible reconstruction has ranged from "What's the point?" to "Don't be so narcissistic," to "What's the matter with falsies . . . You gals have been fooling us for years with them." I'm sure you've come across that kind of response yourself at some time or another.
>
> All this is preamble to a request. Would you be good enough to share your thoughts and your experience with me? I'd really appreciate it if you could. I am determined that no matter what the future has in store, I will do what I can to feel "whole" again if it is at all feasible.

Mrs. C. called to say she was about to go into the hospital for her second mastectomy and was eager to know more about reconstruction. She was hoping to be able to save the nipple from this breast to be divided in half and used on both sides later on. The thought of reconstruction was what was giving her strength for this second battle with cancer.

Mrs. K., widowed for the past ten years, had had a mastectomy a year ago. Last week she had gone to bed for the first time with a man she cared for a great deal. He had proved impotent. She was sure that her disfigured body was the problem. Could she come see me and talk about reconstruction?

Miss G. had seen the *Times* article reprinted in a Chicago paper. She had had a breast removed in December and thought her life was over. But now she had just made an appointment with a plastic surgeon and wanted to tell me she felt as if she had been born again.

Mrs. D., against her husband's, her family doctor's and her surgeon's better judgment, was planning to have only a lumpectomy (removal of the tumor). She wanted to come see me. Maybe she would change her mind after she saw what a reconstruction looked like.

Miss F. had been engaged for the past year and her family had planned an elaborate wedding for June. In January she had lost a breast. She wanted to call off the marriage; her fiancé wanted to go ahead. She was so depressed she had thought of suicide. Could she see me? Maybe there was hope after all.

Miss J. was to have a mastectomy the next week and possibly a prophylactic mastectomy of the other breast (removal of the breast tissue and insertion of an implant under the skin to forestall the possibility of cancer). She had seen photographs of reconstructions and was distressed by the artificial look and the scarring. Maybe if she saw how I looked . . .

Jane R. called for her sister Gladys, thirty-three, who had lost her right breast two years earlier. Gladys was still on chemotherapy, depressed and discouraged. Her husband had left her after the operation. Jane was urging her to have reconstruction.

She thought that would encourage her to meet people, date again, perhaps remarry. When the sisters came to see me, it was hard to decide which one was more miserable—Gladys, because of her loss; Jane, because of her concern for Gladys. They left a lot happier, both pleased with what a new breast looked like and full of plans for finding a plastic surgeon.

A woman came with her lover, a man who said straight out to me, "I like women with two breasts." He had been urging her to have reconstruction; she had balked at any more surgery or hospitals. "I won't undress in front of him any more," she whispered to me when I pulled up my sweater to let her see a reconstructed breast. He looked, too, and when they left, I was sure she was giving second thoughts to her refusal to face more surgery.

A husband and wife came together, very dressy, self-conscious people. "Please let's go into the next room and show me," she asked. He did not ask to look. But when she cried—with happiness at the possibility that opened before her—he cried, too.

A woman who had lost one breast seven years earlier and the other four years after that, phoned me from a hospital in Boston. She was there for her first implant. "Just think," she exulted, "pretty soon I'll be wearing tanksuits again, T-shirts. I'll have breasts."

Quite a number of women told me about the negative attitude of the surgeons they'd consulted. "What are you making such a fuss about?" the leading breast surgeon in a Midwest city asked a patient who was desperately unhappy about her loss. "It isn't as if I'd cut off your arm." Another prominent surgeon deliberately turned his back on a woman when she began to ask him about reconstruction. Another, also questioned about reconstruction, told the patient sharply, "Go home and thank God you're alive."

From these accounts and others similar to them, I realized how much educational work still has to be done among doctors to tune them into the terrible emotional impact of the loss of a breast and the depth of a woman's suffering.

Some doctors even have to be tuned into basic facts about cancer. I was shocked when a woman told me that her husband, a doctor, called her surgeon to ask if it was safe to sleep with her—would he run some risk of "catching" cancer? Maybe some medical schools don't care whom they give degrees to.

A recent letter from a woman in the South underlined the need to make simple, factual information about reconstruction more widely available. This woman wrote:

"I had radical surgery in 1975, when I was thirty-nine, and since then I have tried every kind of bra and prosthesis and still I am miserable all the time. My doctor told me all along there was nothing that could be done as far as surgery, but when I went for a checkup two weeks ago, I told him about an article I had read and asked if I could have this new rebuilding surgery. He said he believes I am cured of cancer and can have the surgery. He put me in touch with a plastic surgeon in the state capital.

"I will appreciate any encouragement you can give. I have been through a state of depression that has affected my whole family, my husband, my fifteen-year-old son and my ten-year-old-daughter. But I am not telling you anything you do not already know."

Several times I visited women in the hospital when they had their reconstruction done. One of them told me her ten-year-old son had said excitedly, "Mommy, Mommy, I can see the bump."

Another, who had been in the depths of despair only a few weeks earlier, was propped up on lacy pillows, writing the outline of a lecture she expected to give to tell other women about reconstruction.

I saw a woman who had had both a breast surgeon and a plastic surgeon in attendance at her mastectomy four days earlier. The former had removed the diseased breast, the latter had stitched the healthy nipple into her groin for future use. "I've got a bad bandage here," she said, pointing to her breast, "and a good one there," and she pointed downward. "It's wonderful to have something positive to look forward to."

Not all my encounters were upbeat. A few days after she came to see me and decided to do reconstruction, Helen K. found a lump on the other side. A second mastectomy uncovered heavy involvement of the lymph nodes. Now she has to defer rebuilding until she finishes her course of chemotherapy. But the thought of reconstruction helps sustain her.

A woman in her fifties had severe radiation burns from x-ray treatment following mastectomy a dozen years earlier. Two plastic surgeons had told her she would need a series of three or four operations to graft tissue from her abdomen to her breast area to form a pocket for an implant. She was triply depressed: by the breast loss, by the heavy scarring and by the obstacles to reconstruction. I know I disappointed her, but I had no happy news for her. For her condition, reconstruction would be complicated and costly.

The calls for help are still coming in. Sometimes I do my show-and-tell a dozen times a week. There is an extraordinary outpouring of emotion in the course of each visit. These women bare their breasts figuratively as I bare mine literally; they tell me wrenching stories of husbands who turn away at their time of greatest need, of lovers—even married lovers—who stand by them, of dashed hopes, of regrets for opportunities not seized, of fears that death is about to touch them.

Conversation

AMY

Amy is a high school principal in Oregon. Her husband is an insurance executive. She is fifty-five, and she had her mastectomy six months ago.

When did you first hear about reconstruction?
I'd read about it and heard it talked about, so as soon as my doctor told me I needed a biopsy, I was already thinking about reconstruction. It was on my mind from the beginning. I'm not sure, but I may not have consented to the surgery if I hadn't had knowledge of reconstruction.

Did you bank the nipple?
No, and I'm very regretful about that. The surgeon didn't suggest it, and while I knew about reconstruction, I didn't know enough to ask to have the nipple saved.

Did your surgeon do a horizontal incision—the kind that makes reconstruction easier?
He wanted to, if possible, but the location of the lesion ruled it out. But, of course, I'm going ahead with the reconstruction. The surgeon says I can have it done in about two months, but I can't wait. I simply hate wearing the prosthesis on the outside. It's not porous and it gathers perspiration underneath and I just can't stand looking at myself. It's going to be interesting because the plastic surgeon will augment my natural breast. He says he has to do that to get symmetry and a good match on both sides. I never wore a bra before the mastectomy and I'm going to be so happy to give up the bra with the prosthesis in it.

What about the nipple?

I haven't quite decided. The surgeon has suggested that he divide the good nipple, but I'm a little worried because I don't want to lose sensitivity in the nipple. That's very important to me, and if it's divided I understand I may lose sensitivity. So I may decide on a labial transplant.

How does your husband feel about reconstruction?

He's all for it. He's not pushing me into it or anything like that. But he's for it because it means so much to me.

And your friends?

That's a funny thing, because as I speak to friends who've had breast surgery and suggest to them that they might be interested in reconstruction, I find they're very reluctant to do anything. These are mostly women in their fifties and I'm amazed by the extent to which they've given up on themselves, on their attractiveness, on their sexuality. It's as if it's all over for them. I really don't understand that attitude. I have a definite purpose in wanting reconstruction. I want to have a second breast because I want to look a lot better than I do now. If you want to say I'm doing it for cosmetic reasons, that's all right with me. I'm not afraid of the word "vanity." And I'm definitely interested in sex.

I think women in their middle years need to do a lot of reevaluation about themselves and their roles. They have to come out and face their sexuality. It's absurd for them to act as if their lives were over. You know, just the other day I was talking about reconstruction with a woman I know who lost her breast quite a number of years go. She said, "What do I need with cleavage at my age? I'm fifty-seven." But she had streaked hair—you know, blond with parts of it much blonder. It seems to me we ought to be more honest with ourselves.

9

The History of Reconstruction

I had originally thought that my reconstruction would end my preoccupation with breasts and breast problems, but the exact opposite was taking place. Every day, as I talked to more and more women, I became more deeply involved in the medical and emotional aspects of breast loss. I even began to wonder about the history of breast replacement.

"Is it really a new idea or has it been going on for quite a while?" I asked Dr. Hoffman one day. He gave me a copy of a paper he had written entitled "Reconstruction of the Female Breast Following Mastectomy." I read it and later I spent some time in the library of the New York Academy of Medicine, digging among the books and periodicals.

I was surprised to learn that the ancient Egyptians, way back in Cleopatra's day, had devised operations to reduce the size of overlarge breasts. I remembered then from courses in ancient history that the Amazons, that legendary race of superwomen, had deliberately amputated their right breast to enhance their skill at bow-and-arrow warfare. If the breast was in the way of ready-aim-fire, off with it, was the attitude of these no-nonsense ladies. Obviously, there was also a strong measure of psychosexual symbolism involved. But, though I wasn't inclined to go into the self-image problems of ancient warrior women, I couldn't help wondering whether any individual

Amazon had ever lamented her severed breast and longed for its recovery.

I discovered that reconstruction as we know it today dates back just under a century. Anyone who reads the old records can only marvel at the courage and stamina of the handful of pioneer women who underwent the complicated, often gruesome and frankly experimental surgery of the late nineteenth century. How fierce must have been their drive to achieve wholeness again—in an era when plastic surgery was barely in its infancy and all surgery was fraught with terrible danger!

Despite the odds against them, a few women persisted and a few surgeons dared. In 1887 an unsung heroine allowed a Dr. Verneuil, a French surgeon, to use part of her healthy breast to rebuild the diseased one after a malignancy was removed. Fifteen years later another French surgeon, a Dr. Morestin, found a way after a mastectomy to divide the remaining breast in two and used half of it for the reconstruction. A few other surgeons around the turn of the century attempted to fashion a new breast out of part of the remaining one. But the technique met with so little success that the cases on record are regarded as medical oddities.

Hardly more successful were early efforts to transplant tissue from elsewhere on the woman's body to the breast area. A surgeon named Czerny tried transplanting a benign fatty tumor called a lipoma from a patient's back to the breast area. About the time of World War I several German surgeons switched fatty deposits from various parts of the body to the breast. The basic trouble with this procedure was that the body tended to absorb the fat and the new breast gradually melted away.

The first step toward successful breast reconstruction came with the development of what plastic surgeons call a pedicle flap. This is a piece of tissue partially cut away from one part of the body, but left with an attachment at its original location which provides a blood supply. The free end of the flap is then grafted to the part of the body where the new tissue is wanted. As soon as the graft "takes" and the tissue is being adequately nourished in its new location, the pedicle is cut away and reattached in the new area.

More complicated versions of the pedicle flap may require several steps. For example, there was the case of a thirteen-year-old girl who never developed a left breast because of heavy x-ray doses in infancy. A pedicle flap was made from her right buttock to her right forearm—which meant that the flap linked the forearm to the buttock area for several weeks. Then the pedicle was cut away from the buttock and sewn to the chest wall on the left side. This time the flap was being nourished from its attachment to the right wrist, which had to remain close to the breast area until the breast end of the flap "took." At that stage the pedicle was cut away from the wrist and sewn to the chest to form a pocket into which a silicone implant was inserted.

This example illustrates a very modern application of the pedicle technique, but it enabled me to visualize the process so vividly that I pass it along here to help you form a clear picture in your mind of what is meant by a pedicle flap, or, as it is often called simply, a flap.

At any rate, one of the first recorded uses of a flap to re-create a breast was tried by Kleinschmidt, a German surgeon, in 1924. Then in 1945 a British surgeon cut away a fatty fold across a patient's rather ample abdomen, but left this tissue attached to her body at both ends. He sewed together the top and bottom edges of what he had cut away to form a tube and pulled together the edges left on her body and sewed them up to make a tighter, flatter tummy. After the seam along the tube had healed, he cut away one end of the tube and sewed it into an opening he'd made in the area of the missing breast. Still later, the other end of the tube was moved up to the chest, and after that the tube was molded into a breastlike shape. By 1956 Dr. B. S. Freeman was using the tube technique to transfer in stages half of a large breast to form a new one on the other side.

Dr. Millard, at the University of Miami School of Medicine, tried an abdominal flap for breast reconstruction for the first time in 1957. Unfortunately, the flap included an old appendectomy scar, which created so many complications that half of the new breast failed. The surgeon had to start over with more flaps and then use a flap from the flank to repair the area cut away from the abdomen. In this case he reconstructed an areola and nipple from the umbilicus or navel, which he everted, or turned inside out. Despite all that she went through, the patient was satisfied with her new breast. In fact, she had only one complaint—the loss of her navel. So the surgeon obligingly created an umbilical dimple for her.

You can see the disadvantages of flap transplants—they take time, require many operations and leave scars both on the donor site and in the reconstructed area. But they are still in use in special circumstances. One of these is reconstruction after a radical mastectomy in which the pectoral muscle has been removed and the skin is heavily scarred by radiation or when radiation damage has already been repaired by skin grafts. Flap transplants are *not* necessary for breast reconstruction after most modified mastectomies. As the use of the radical mastectomy declines, so will the need for this reconstruction technique.

What has really made modern breast reconstruction possible, of course, is the silicone implant. Earlier implants, made of various plastics, had a way of forming hard mounds. Often the mound would shrink and turn lumpy. Patients complained that after all the trouble they'd gone to, they ended up with a breast that resembled a baseball or, in extreme cases, a golf ball. Then, in the early 1960s Dr. Thomas Cronin and Dr. F. J. Gerow of Houston, Texas, developed a silicone prosthesis for use in operations to enlarge undersized breasts.

As augmentation mammoplasty became increasingly popular—not just for fan dancers but for thousands of women discontented with their natural endowments—the silicone implants got better and better. They became available in a variety of sizes and shapes. Some consisted of a silicone envelope inflated with a saline solution after implantation. Others contained a silicone gel. Refinements included inner compartments that allowed the gel to float within the outer envelope in order to simulate the movement of a natural breast.

One of the first reports in the medical literature of a silicone implant used for reconstruction described the work of Dr. Reuben Snyderman and Dr. Randolph Guthrie at New York Hospital in 1970. These surgeons made a horizontal incision low on the patient's chest and slid a small prosthesis upward between the skin and the chest wall.

A few years later surgeons tried a vertical incision at the underarm side of the breast and inserted the implant from the side. They found this type of operation helpful in maintaining blood supply to the thinly stretched skin over the implant. This is the operation that Dr. Hoffman performed for me in 1974.

There were two things wrong with the new breast created by the insertion of a silicone implant: it was usually smaller and rounder than the remaining breast, and it lacked a nipple.

But the ingenuity of the plastic surgeons was equal to the situation on both counts. Breast reduction as a cosmetic procedure had become almost as popular as breast augmentation. The same surgeons who were just beginning to build new breasts had already established long records of success at scaling down overlarge, pendulous and flabby breasts. Now they put this known technique to work for their reconstruction patients and reshaped the healthy but too ample or sagging real breast to match the youthfully rounded replacement on the other side.

That's what happened to me and I've already described my surprise and delight at recapturing the firm natural uplift of my teen years.

As for the nipple, efforts to reconstruct it have followed many paths. More than fifty years ago Dr. Kleinschmidt, that imaginative German pioneer, tried to simulate a nipple by cutting away a circle of skin in the appropriate place with the hope that the resulting scar would look a little like a nipple. It didn't really. Some doctors gathered up a bit of skin, again in the appropriate place, and whipped surgical thread around it to form a protuberance. No luck.

The inside-out umbilicus had its advocates and worked after

a fashion when the breast was rebuilt with abdominal tissue.

In 1949 Dr. W. M. Adams described in the *Journal of Plastic and Reconstructive Surgery* his method of using a graft from the labia minor, the inner folds near the vagina, to construct an areola. The tissue matched the areola reasonably well in color, and the transplant was so thin that it could be attached as a free graft, directly from one site to another without the intermediate step of flaps to maintain circulation. Today the labial graft is in standard usage, with some surgeons preferring the labia major, or outer lips, as a source and others favoring the labia minor. Sometimes a doctor uses the major for the areola and the minor for the nipple.

Tattooing has had its advocates and there are still some surgeons who use it. Unfortunately, an areola created by tattooing the area to a reddish tint tends to fade. The failure, however, may lie more in the tattooer than in the process itself. Even the best of plastic surgeons is not a very skilled tattoo artist. Who knows—perhaps if some hospital were to employ an old tattoo hand from Hawaii who's spent a lifetime applying supergraphics to sailors' chests and biceps, the tattooed areola might become a big success.

Another approach is the fashioning of a nipple and areola from a part of the remaining normal nipple. This technique was tried as far back as 1923 by a Dr. Aubert, a French surgeon. It works especially well when the remaining nipple-areola complex is large and when the division is done at the time the healthy breast is being reduced in size to match the rebuilt one. Nipple-sharing techniques have been so refined that the plastic surgeon has about half a dozen to choose from. He may transplant the lower half of the remaining nipple-areola, move concentric circles of the tissue, make an S-like division of the tissue or even a complicated pinwheel sharing.

The idea of banking the nipple of the amputated breast was urged by Dr. Millard on his plastic surgeon colleagues as early as 1971. In an editorial in the *American Journal of Surgery* he pointed out that when the nipple is saved and sewn into a woman's groin for future use, it serves as a "token of her doctor's faith in her cure and eventual rehabilitation."

One surgeon has reported the case of a woman whose nipple was sewn into her groin at the time of her mastectomy. When the day came for her reconstruction, this patient backed away, explaining that she'd made a satisfactory adjustment to her single-breasted state. No, she didn't want to bother removing the banked nipple—she didn't want any more surgery of any kind, thank you.

One date I would like very much to record but have not been able to pinpoint—surely it was within the last half dozen years —is the first time a cancer surgeon and a plastic surgeon cooperated in planning a patient's reconstruction. That, indeed, was a historic occasion. By 1972 cooperation, or at least the idea of cooperation, had advanced to the point that a symposium was held on "Problems of the Female Breast" at Memorial Sloan-Kettering Cancer Center in New York City, jointly sponsored by Memorial Hospital, the world-famous cancer institution, and the Educational Foundation of the American Society of Plastic and Reconstructive Surgeons. Described as a "milestone in interdisciplinary exploration," the symposium brought together general surgeons, breast surgeons, plastic surgeons, pathologists and radiologists.

The tone of the meeting was highly favorable to reconstruction. "Plastic surgeons will in the future be deeply and increasingly involved in the treatment of breast problems," declared Dr. Snyderman, who edited the proceedings of the symposium for a book published in 1973 by C. V. Mosby Company.

As I continued to delve into the history of reconstruction, a strange thing happened. The more I read and learned, the angrier I got. I myself had stumbled onto reconstruction in 1974 through my own persistent searchings. At that time the idea seemed far-out, even ridiculous, to the people I met and to most of the doctors I talked to. My own plastic surgeon had done only a handful of reconstructions. I'd never met a woman who had a rebuilt breast. There was no word of this procedure in the popular press.

Yet all through the first half of the 1970s there had been

dozens and dozens of articles in reputable medical publications reporting favorably on breast reconstruction. Diagrams, drawings and photographs of successful reconstructions were being displayed at the national conventions of plastic surgeons. As far back as 1972 many of the country's outstanding practitioners in cancer surgery and in plastic surgery had gotten together to discuss reconstruction among other breast problems. Their findings had been published and made available to other doctors.

How come, then, that I had not been told about breast reconstruction when I asked and asked and asked?

Maybe I'm unrealistically impatient. Maybe I just don't understand a snail's pace. But it does seem odd to me that in view of (1) the many efforts at breast reconstruction which have been going on in various parts of the world all through this decade of the seventies; (2) the many successes that have been recorded in the medical literature; (3) the diverse techniques that have been developed in the past decade; and (4) the degree of cooperation that has already been achieved at the highest level between cancer surgeons and plastic surgeons—in view of all this, the possibility of reconstruction is still a carefully kept secret from most of the ninety thousand women a year who undergo mastectomy.

10

The State of the Controversy

One reason for the secrecy about breast reconstruction might be that the surgery is still too controversial to be made generally available. But I reject that answer. I reject it because I am convinced that reconstruction is one of the least controversial aspects of the whole breast cancer problem today.

The big debate now taking place among doctors and informed—and, perhaps, not-so-informed—lay people centers on the best management of the disease itself.

A dozen years ago the maximum amount of surgery was considered the only acceptable treatment for breast cancer. Today there are highly articulate advocates of a variety of different approaches. In fact, the intense debate over the extent of surgery necessary for optimal results has led many surgeons to perform fewer of the disfiguring radical operations and more of the less drastic modified radicals.

A few surgeons now even favor lumpectomy in appropriate cases and argue that their cure rate from taking out only the lump and leaving the rest of the breast is as good as that obtained by more extensive surgery.

Radiologists who use intensive radiation and temporary cobalt implants, without surgery or with removal only of the diseased tissue, make strong claims for their high cure rates.

Proponents of prophylactic mastectomy make assertions

about the merit of their procedure which are disputed and questioned by others.

The long-running debate about how much radiation, if any, to give following mastectomy has been pretty much resolved in favor of no radiation. Chemotherapy is the treatment of choice when the lymph nodes are involved. But there is an ongoing discussion about the most effective combination of drugs and duration of treatment with chemotherapy.

No wonder that a team of Harvard researchers recently characterized breast cancer treatment as the most highly controversial area in medicine today.

Meanwhile, extreme feminists are proclaiming that mastectomy is a brutal male ploy against females. Less extreme feminists and women who don't consider themselves feminists at all are demanding a stronger role in deciding how much, if any, of their bodies is to be cut away. Thousands of women are routinely rejecting the fatherly pat on the knee by the all-knowing surgeon and insisting on learning precisely what choices are possible and what advantages and disadvantages accompany each avenue of treatment.

There are even angry attacks on the whole cancer establishment for failing to reduce the mortality from breast cancer in the last forty years and allowing it to continue as the number one cancer killer of women.

You can tune in on the pros and cons of the great breast cancer debate in the medical press, the popular press, the feminist press, on television talk shows, at medical meetings, in the publications of various cancer organizations and agencies.

While this debate rages, reconstruction moves forward—virtually without debate.

In the outline of this book submitted to the publisher I proposed a chapter on the controversy over reconstruction. I was sure there must be important voices of dissent that should be heard, and it would not be fair to report only favorable views. I wanted to give equal time and space to opponents of reconstruction.

With a few, very limited exceptions, I haven't been able to find much controversy. Whatever doubt may have existed in the past about the safety and propriety of breast reconstruction pretty much vanished early in 1977, when the American Cancer Society, Inc., distributed a circular to doctors and health care agencies around the country entitled "Statement Re: Reconstructive Surgery After Mastectomy." The statement reads as follows:

> Upon recommendation of the National Task Force on Breast Cancer, the Society's Board of Directors at its meeting on February 4, 1977, approved the following statement on Reconstructive Surgery After Mastectomy:
>
> "Rehabilitation is an integral part of the management of the patient with breast cancer. The Society's interest has been successfully expressed primarily through the Reach to Recovery Program which provides psychological, physical and cosmetic rehabilitation to the mastectomy patient. This does not preclude reconstructive efforts in suitable instances.
>
> "The basic thrust of the physician should be to improve cure and survival. When this can be accomplished without prejudicing the prospects of physical reconstruction, every effort should be made to preserve a suitable physical base for such restoration.
>
> "The Society will continue to expand its educational programs so that both physicians and patients may be aware of the potentials of reconstructive surgery. This does not diminish the importance of the Reach to Recovery Program, but may well serve as an additional measure in appropriate instances to improve the quality of survival."
>
> It was noted that this is fundamentally an issue to be decided by the responsible general surgeon, the patient and the plastic surgeon. However, it was agreed that the Society should have available a uniform statement in response to inquiries from the public.

That statement serves in many ways as a turning point in the history of reconstruction by giving it the stamp of approval of the powerful, prestigious and notably conservative American Cancer Society. The society is not known to favor dubious cures or questionable treatments. On the contrary, it is frequently under attack for withholding endorsement of cancer-management practices that have their specialized and often highly vocal supporters.

With its statement that clearly accepts reconstruction, the society has ended most debate over the risk of restorative surgery. The society's medical experts are obviously convinced that the rebuilding of an amputated breast will not put the patient in jeopardy in terms of cancer.

If anyone needs further assurance, there is the fact that reconstructions are performed regularly and without special fanfare at Memorial Sloan-Kettering Cancer Center in New York, at the hospitals of leading medical centers across the country and at teaching hospitals of major medical schools. This operation is not, and never has been, the kind that is performed furtively in back rooms.

Dr. Jerome Urban of Memorial says, "I do support the reconstructive procedure wherever possible. It is an incentive to some women to come early for cancer diagnosis. I understand very well the great relief it provides for mastectomy patients."

Dr. Roy Ashikari, chief of the Breast Service clinic at Memorial, says, "Cancer is our common enemy. But I have no objection to reconstruction. It does not stir up recurrence of the cancer. If the cancer is one centimeter or less in diameter, I want the woman to wait one year for reconstruction. If the cancer is bigger than one centimeter, I want her to wait two years. It is important to remember that we have to treat not only the cancer but the woman, too."

What about the implant? Is the silicone a potential source of trouble? Dr. Hoffman says, "At this time there is no correlation between silicone and cancer."

Silicone has been implanted in the human body for the past fifteen years without harmful effect, not just for breast rebuilding but for many types of reconstructive surgery and as the casing of hundreds of thousands of cardiac pacemakers as well. Whether there will be negative findings in twenty or thirty years remains to be seen. What can be said now is that there is no hint or indication of difficulties ahead.

(I'd like to repeat once more that we are *not* talking about injection of liquid silicone, a technique tried with dire results some years ago for the enlargement of undersized breasts. Not only did the silicone migrate away from the breast area, it also invaded other tissues and led to a number of fatalities before its use was banned by some states.)

If you're wondering if an implant might mask the development of a future cancer, I should tell you at this point that I have a mammogram every twelve months of *both* breasts. My doctor advises me that the mammogram is able to pick up changes in the underlayers of the skin covering the implant and in the tissue between the implant and the chest wall. The scar of the mastectomy incision, although greatly faded, is still visible and easily inspected for thickening or suspicious changes.

Dr. Milton T. Edgerton, head of plastic surgery at the University of Virginia Hospital, points out another positive aspect of reconstruction. "Whenever we do a reconstruction at this hospital," he explains, "we biopsy the tissue on the chest wall before we insert the implant. That means the reconstruction patient gets a little extra measure of protection that is not generally available to the woman who has undergone mastectomy."

None of this is to say that every breast cancer surgeon is wildly enthusiastic about breast reconstruction. I'm sure that some, perhaps many, have their reservations, spoken or unspoken. One doctor who voices his is, as we have noted, Dr. C. D. Haagensen, of Columbia Presbyterian Hospital in New York.

Dr. Haagensen told me, "I disapprove of breast reconstructions following mastectomy for breast cancer. They fail aesthetically, but even more important, they are dangerous. If you have cancer left on the chest wall, the reconstructive operation may spread the cancer around. What's more, the larger the foreign body in the human body [he was referring to the breast implant], the greater the danger of infection."

Dr. Haagensen does *only* radical mastectomies. He does not approve of the less disfiguring modified mastectomies that in recent years have become the operation of choice among many breast cancer surgeons when the patient's condition permits this lesser surgery. Dr. Haagensen claims that because of his radical operation his cure rate is 10 percent higher than the prevailing survival figures for the less thorough modified mastectomy.

When I told him of my own satisfactory experience with reconstruction, he replied, "I don't deprecate your personal experience, but breast cancer is a very dangerous disease. The most complete and thorough operation is the safest. There is a great tendency to do incomplete operations which permit doing a reconstruction later."

Dr. Haagensen undoubtedly has some colleagues who share his distrust of reconstruction. But among leading cancer surgeons his is the only voice of dissent that reaches the public. And in my wide reading of medical periodicals and texts, and in my interviews with surgeons, I did not find any other opponent of breast reconstruction after mastectomy. Some skeptics, yes, especially among cancer surgeons, as to whether women really care that much about having two breasts. ("Yes, Doctor, they do!") But no surgeons predicting dire consequences of reconstruction.

On the contrary, many cancer surgeons welcome reconstruction, not only for its aesthetic value and the emotional lift it imparts, but also for the impetus it gives women to overcome their terror of mutilation and to act promptly at the first sign of a breast problem.

So much, then, for controversy.

11

The Current State of the Art: Routine Procedures

Obviously, all the medical facts and surgical procedures discussed in this book have been checked for accuracy—by at least one and sometimes by two qualified physicians. Two of the chapters most carefully checked were this and the following one, which tell women about the various kinds of breast reconstruction surgery available today.

The surgeon who reviewed the material in this chapter suggested the title. "These are really routine procedures," he said, "so why don't you call the chapter that?"

I really liked his suggestion. Routine. What a reassuring word. Brushing your teeth. Putting out the cat. Setting the breakfast table the night before. Isn't it fascinating that a plastic surgeon thinks of certain kinds of breast rebuilding as routine? We really have come a long way.

To start at the beginning, the most widely performed reconstruction is the type I had which involves the creation of a pocket under the skin and the insertion of an implant shaped like a breast. The implants most generally used come in a number of sizes, but the choice of size is less related to the dimensions of the original breast than to the amount of skin available to form a cover over the insert. Sometimes only a very small implant can be used at the beginning. Then later, when the skin stretches out a bit, the incision can be reopened and a larger mound placed in the pocket.

Depending on the surgeon who performs the operation, the incision for the implant may be vertical or horizontal. A few surgeons may reopen the mastectomy incision for implant insertion, but this is not the common practice.

Dr. Hoffman prefers a vertical incision on the side of the chest below the axilla (armpit) because he thinks it interferes less with the vital blood supply to the skin of the breast area. (The vertical incision somewhat resembles an old-fashioned side placket on a dress.)

Dr. Randolph Guthrie of New York Hospital, on the other hand, favors a horizontal incision just under the breast for precisely the same reason—preservation of circulation.

Dr. Hoffman also likes the vertical incision because he finds he can slightly loosen the skin of the back behind the incision and pull it forward so as to provide a little extra fullness in the breast region.

Dr. Guthrie says the skin of the back is relatively inelastic, and the vertical incision sometimes requires a skin graft to close up the gap. Dr. Hoffman says he rarely uses a skin graft with the vertical incision.

The horizontal incision usually coincides with the natural skin fold under the breast and is therefore not very noticeable. The vertical scar is slightly visible.

Both surgeons get excellent results with their differing methods, and I cite both in detail to show you that surgeons' judgments differ.

Whatever the incision, what goes inside is a silicone envelope which may contain silicone gel or a saline solution, depending on the preference of the surgeon. The surface of the prosthesis containing a gel may have a roughened texture so that it will "grow" into the subcutaneous tissue and remain in the proper position. The surface of the saline prosthesis has a smooth texture. Earlier implants tended to wrinkle, so that the breast sometimes looked like a badly stuffed pillow. That defect has been improved on.

A reconstruction of this type takes about an hour, is done in the hospital, usually under general anesthesia, requires a hospital stay of two to four days, a few days of restricted activity afterwards and perhaps a touch more than the normal caution in avoiding a blow to the breast.

What can go wrong? Occasionally an infection occurs after the operation. Occasionally there is an impairment of circulation and the skin may not tolerate the presence of the implant under it. The implant may have to be removed immediately, or the skin over the implant may slough away and the implant may extrude through the skin. If this happens, the operation may be redone.

Another problem is contracture. The scar around the implant, particularly the inner scar where subsurface tissues have been cut and then must heal, may shrink to the extent that the silicone is squeezed into a rigid hard breast. This is not a frequent occurrence (it seems to happen more often in breast augmentation than in reconstruction), but if it does take place, the scar tissue can sometimes be released. Unfortunately, it may not always stay released.

Some women are a little disappointed because the implant is somewhat firmer than the natural breast. My implant was quite firm at the outset, but it has softened considerably over a three-year period and now is fairly close to the density of my other breast.

Dr. Shattuck W. Hartwell, Jr., of the Cleveland Clinic in Ohio, recently reported on twenty-one reconstructions performed in a ten-year period. One patient, for unknown reasons, asked for the removal of the implant soon after insertion; one had a breakdown of the skin after six years; and one had drainage through the nipple after ten years, which necessitated removal. All the rest were successful.

Commenting on the failures, Dr. Hartwell said, "The most common complication may be a dissatisfied patient." According to him, dissatisfaction may result from an error in judgment on the part of the surgeon or a failure to assess the suitability of the available remaining skin and muscle, or from inadequate preparation of the patient as to what to expect.

In most cases today the nipple and areola are created with the use of labial tissue around the vagina. Some doctors do this as an office procedure, others in the hospital. Nipple sharing (dividing the good nipple) has its advocates, especially when the remaining nipple is large and the remaining breast is being reduced. In that case, the nipple-areola often needs to be reduced in size, too, to maintain proper proportions, so it's simple enough to use some of the excess tissue on the other side.

If, however, the remaining breast does not need to be conformed to the newly built one, most women, understandably, are reluctant to cut into the good nipple when the labial transplant is easily available.

As for nipple banking, there, if anywhere, you find somewhat different ideas. Dr. Urban says, "At times there is some danger involved, since the nipple may contain Paget's cells—a form of breast cancer. This occurs in about three percent of patients with breast cancer." He prefers nipple reconstruction from the labia or the opposite nipple.

"However, in some cases, the nipple can be banked when the nipple and areola are made very thin, and the underlying tissue has been reviewed by the pathologist at the time of the original surgery," he says.

Dr. Guy Robbins, of Sloan-Kettering, goes even further than Dr. Urban in his opposition. He says of nipple banking, "It's crazy. There are ducts in the nipple that may contain breast cancer." Some plastic surgeons are not very much impressed with this objection because they routinely remove the ducts in the nipple before it is banked.

Dr. Robert M. Goldwyn, a prominent plastic surgeon in Boston, says, "I have not used nipple banking because the general surgeons with whom I work at Harvard Medical School prefer not to use the nipple and areola from a breast which has had cancer or severe premalignant disease."

Other surgeons, however, approve of nipple banking provided the tumor is small, it is located far away from the nipple, the nipple itself is disease-free and biopsies taken from underneath the nipple are negative. Sometimes the cancer surgeon stitches the nipple to the place where it is to be temporarily stored. At other times the plastic surgeon is present at the mastectomy and takes care of the nipple banking.

What saves the nipple-reconstruction situation, no matter how it is done, is the extraordinary range in size, shape, projection and coloration of the nipple-areola complex. Not only are all these variations normal, but it often happens that there is a marked difference between a woman's right and left nipples.

If you ever go to a sauna or a health club where large numbers of women walk around with their breasts exposed, you can't help observing all the variations in nipples. The first time you may even have trouble keeping from staring. As a result, the nipple built by the plastic surgeon can be considered good, even if it does not conform totally to the woman's natural nipple. In my own case, the reconstructed nipple is flatter and slightly darker than the natural nipple, but no one seems to notice.

A reconstructed nipple is not erectile and lacks sensitivity to sexual stimulation. This is unavoidable, since the mammary nerves were removed in the mastectomy and the new nipple's only connection is to the skin around it. Nevertheless, a number of women have confided to me that the rebuilt nipple has, with time, developed some sensitivity. Who really knows whether erogenous reactions originate on the skin or in the head? Sensitivity is not impaired in the labial area where tissue was removed, and the incision is so small there is virtually no scarring.

As for the need to reduce the other breast, that will depend on the breast's size and the woman's expectation of what reconstruction will offer. If the breast she lost was small and high, the reconstruction may closely resemble the real thing. If so, the lucky patient needs no further correction.

In many cases, however, the lost breast has already sagged or dropped to some extent. At the present state of the art, surgeons are not able to sculpt a new breast with a downward swoop. Neither can they construct an ample breast under the remaining skin that is tightly drawn across the chest wall. The patient who is satisfied to regain a sense of wholeness, recapture some degree of cleavage and look reasonably presentable in a bra may be able to ignore either minor or major imbalance from left to right.

On the other hand, if symmetry is important and the woman wants to be able to look at herself nude in the mirror, she will have to undergo the procedure known as reduction mammoplasty or mastopexy, which is breast reduction with nipple relocation to a position higher up on the curve of the breast.

Both these operations are frequently done by plastic surgeons for patients who elect them for aesthetic reasons totally unrelated to cancer. They are performed in the hospital, under general anesthesia, require three days of hospitalization and usually leave a horizontal scar under the curve of the breast and a vertical scar from the base of the breast to the nipple. Both scars fade in time, but they are permanent and cannot be removed.

One type of breast that gives the surgeon a certain amount of trouble in reconstruction is the wide, flat, pancake-shaped breast. Implants are not currently made in that shape and must be specially devised for the individual patient. When the breast shape is unusual, some doctors use a technique called moulage, which involves the making of a wax impression and then a plaster cast of the chest area as a guide to the surgeon in his attempt to make the implant conform in size and shape to the other breast.

Sometimes a woman with very small breasts will request an implant somewhat larger than her normal size, if a sufficient pocket can be constructed, and then will undergo breast augmentation surgery on the other side.

12

The Current State of the Art: Complex Procedures

So far we've talked only about the simpler kinds of reconstruction. The task is more complicated if the main chest muscle has been removed or if the skin has been damaged by radiation or patched with a skin graft. In fact, until quite recently it was *extremely* complicated and required a long series of operations and hospitalizations. But now a number of plastic surgeons are finding less complex ways to deal with radical mastectomies.

Dr. Guthrie, for example, who has performed 118 reconstructions since 1970 and is now doing them at a rate of more than 100 a year, uses a special elongated implant to fill in the concave area where the pectoral muscle was removed. A few other surgeons are also using custom-made prostheses to correct the hollow or depression that has been left by extensive surgery.

Why is it so difficult to replace the missing chest muscle? Mobility is the answer. Replacing a breast is relatively easy because the breast is not a very mobile part of the body. True, it moves and flows to the side when you lie down. But otherwise there is not much motion in the breast tissue. So all the rebuilt breast has to do is to *be* there and look and feel to the touch as much like a real breast as possible.

But that area up by the shoulder is different. It is in constant motion when you raise or lower your arm, twist or turn your upper body, bend, reach or turn in bed. A physician or physical therapist will almost certainly recommend exercises, following mastectomy, to restore mobility to the shoulder and upper arm.

But that mobility you need to function normally makes it difficult for whatever reconstruction the surgeon attempts in the hollow where the muscle once was. You certainly don't want an implant that interferes with mobility—you've already had enough interference from the mastectomy itself. The reconstruction must not only look right; it must also work and move well.

That's why even the most ingenious plastic surgeon finds it a great challenge to mimic nature when the muscle and underarm area have to be rebuilt. It also explains why some plastic surgeons are reluctant even to attempt a reconstruction after a radical. But others, after warning a patient of the difficulties ahead, are willing to offer their best efforts.

A leading surgeon in Germany and a handful in this country are using something called omentum in these reconstructions. This is a fatty substance found inside the abdomen which can be moved up to the chest area through a tunnel incision. One end of the omentum remains permanently attached in the abdomen so that it continues to receive nourishment while the main volume of the fatty material serves as replacement for the missing breast.

Most American surgeons see little value in moving omentum around, since silicone implants are so readily available, but a few do find omentum useful in rebuilding chest walls damaged by radiation burns and in filling in hollowed areas after radicals.

When there is radiation damage or a previous skin graft to correct an x-ray burn, or when the skin is too tight or thin to cover an implant, the most generally available procedure is still the multi-step flap that requires at least three operations to get the flap up to the chest area from the abdomen, flank or buttock and usually two more to construct the breast.

In a paper presented to the annual meeting of the American Society of Plastic and Reconstruction Surgeons in 1975 in Toronto, Canada, Dr. Millard told his colleagues that patients needing flaps should "plan a year for the reconstruction, and maybe more, so that the stages need not be hurried and the tissues have a chance to settle and soften."

Dr. Millard described in detail the reconstruction of a forty-two-year-old woman five years after a radical with heavy scarring on her chest and with recurring cysts in her other breast. He made a tube of excess abdominal tissue that was later transferred in several stages to the mammary area to reinforce the scarred tissue and form a pocket that would house an implant. These steps took ten months. Four months after that, he removed the cystic tissue of the other breast, reduced the breast in size and inserted a silicone gel implant. Later a piece of silicone rubber was shaped to fill the deficiency in the contour of the upper chest where the pectoral muscle had been removed. At the same time, half the good nipple was used to create a prominence in the center of the other side.

What this woman got, after a year and a half of multiple surgeries, was a nice flat abdomen, two shapely symmetrical breasts and a great feeling of satisfaction. Most women would admire her fortitude in pursuing her goals, but only a tiny dedicated minority would be interested in following her footsteps in those repeated visits to the operating room.

Today even the complicated flap procedures are being improved. Some plastic surgeons have found ways to raise a flap from the thoracic area just under the breast. They take skin from the thorax in the triangular shape of an upside-down bikini top (with the point at the bottom), flip it upward over the breast area and attach it above a small silicone implant. An operation of this type is still a virtuoso performance and not to be expected in daily medical practice. However, it indicates the daring and imagination that are now being applied to the correction of breast disfigurement and promises new and better procedures for the future. It should be stressed again that these drastic procedures are needed only when there is severe disfigurement or special problems.

Another operation is the prophylactic subcutaneous mastectomy. The idea is that since the female breast has been described as a cancer factory, why not head off cancer in a breast that seems particularly at risk. In this operation, most of the underlying breast tissue is excised, but the skin is left intact and usually the nipple-areola complex also remains untouched. A silicone implant is inserted, either at the time of the subcutaneous mastectomy or preferably at a later date.

With the removal of tissues that could potentially become cancerous, the threat of malignancy is presumably lifted. Scarring is minimal. And the presence of the woman's own nipple reassures her that her body has not really changed.

Another way to attain the objective of preventing cancer before it occurs is to do a simple mastectomy (removal of the breast but not the lymph nodes or the underlying muscle), followed by reconstruction.

Since either of these prophylactic operations (subcutaneous or simple) is done before cancer strikes, the procedure is not really a cancer operation. For that reason, and also because aesthetic considerations are so important, the breast removal as well as the rebuilding is usually handled by a plastic surgeon.

You may wonder who would go to the extreme of cutting away a noncancerous breast. The women who choose this surgery are, for the most part, at very high risk. They have gone through the trial and suspense of several biopsies, their family histories reveal a proneness to breast cancer and their nerves are frazzled from constant worry about their breasts and about what new lump or thickening may present itself tomorrow or the next day.

Occasionally a subcutaneous or a simple mastectomy is chosen instead of breast reduction by a woman whose remaining breast is being revised to match her rebuilt one. She may make this choice if there is evidence of premalignant disease in the breast or if she is considered at high risk to lose that breast to cancer.

Not every woman who chooses prophylactic mastectomy is happy afterwards. I know one in her thirties who had been plagued with breast problems all her adult life and lived in constant dread of cancer. She chose bilateral subcutaneous mastectomy as soon as she learned about it. But a year later her enthusiasm had drained away. First she had problems with the circulation in the skin over the implants, then one of the implants extruded through the skin and later the skin on one side contracted, squeezing the silicone into a hard ball.

"This whole thing was nothing to rush into," she now says, sadder but wiser. "And if I were to do it again, I'd wait a while between having the breast tissue removed and the insert put in. I've changed surgeons and the new one says it's just too traumatic to the system to do everything all at once on both sides. It isn't reasonable to expect the body to handle all that healing and readjustment at one time."

Dr. Milton Edgerton, at the University of Virginia Hospital, allows an interval of about five days between removing the breast tissue and placing the implant. He finds that even that slight delay greatly improves the chances of success for a subcutaneous mastectomy.

About the only thing worse than having a mastectomy is having two. But there is one small reward for the woman who has undergone this double suffering. She is considered the ideal candidate for reconstruction. The surgeon does not have to worry about matching an implant to the opposite breast in shape, size, density and nipple location. Neither does he have to reduce the natural breast to conform to the rebuilt one. Within the limitations of the skin available, he can position twin implants in identical locations on each side of the chest and lo! a perfect match.

If the bilateral mastectomy was radical, however, the news is not quite so cheerful. The heroic surgery that at this time is the usual method of correcting the defect must be doubled. It is only for the woman with a truly massive need to return her body to wholeness.

There is one question I am repeatedly asked: Why all the delays? If the implant surgery is so easily done, why can't it be performed at the same time as the original mastectomy? That way, there would only be one hospitalization and the patient would awaken with a new breast and skip the entire horror of living, even temporarily, with an amputation.

You can be sure that I've asked quite a number of surgeons that question myself. I've found that one or two surgeons in this country are inserting the implant at the time of the mastectomy, and in Australia there is one surgeon who slips in the prosthesis a few days after the mastectomy through the original incision. But most cancer surgeons and plastic surgeons, too, disapprove strongly of this procedure.

Dr. Hartwell in Cleveland originally did simultaneous reconstructions a decade ago but was not satisfied with the results. He now waits four months after the mastectomy to position the prosthesis and another four weeks to form a nipple. He finds that the two operations are less traumatic to the patient, they allow him to define the pocket more accurately and they assure a better blood supply. In addition, he has discovered that the insert may need an altogether different incision from the one made by the cancer surgeon.

Dr. Hoffman, like most of his colleagues, wants the mastectomy incision to heal completely and soften for six to eight months before attempting another operation. He also points out that it is important to define the placement of the implant while the patient is sitting or standing up, which, of course, cannot be done as well on the operating table.

Dr. Cronin in Texas, who has done reconstructions as early as four days and as late as twenty-five years after mastectomy, prefers a delay of two to three months for both medical and psychological reasons. He thinks a woman is more likely to be satisfied with her not-quite-perfect rebuilt breast if she has lived for a while with a flat, scarred chest.

As to time, there is one remarkable thing about reconstruction—no statute of limitations. Whether the mastectomy was performed one year, ten years or even thirty years in the past, as long as the woman is in good health, is free of cancer and wants her body rebuilt, she can probably have it. Dr. Cronin has told of operating on two sixty-year-old women. One had had a modified radical twenty-seven years earlier and a large biopsy in the other breast. The other had a remaining breast that was pendulous with a nipple at the very bottom. In both cases he rebuilt the breast on the mastectomy side and reshaped the other side to match.

13

The Psychology of Breast Loss

One day it struck me that all the stories I was listening to from women had two aspects—one medical and one emotional.

The medical details of their mastectomies varied considerably. But the emotional content of their narratives was always remarkably similar. Shock, anger, grief, bereavement, depression, despair, hostility, sexual problems, loss of self-esteem, fear.

Some women were so depressed they'd gone into hiding. A few were suicidal at times. Many masked their unhappiness with outward calm or gaiety and then, at some key moment, let the mask fall away to reveal the sheer terror underneath.

What surprised me was that only one woman of the many I talked to had received any kind of support—counseling or therapy from a psychologist, psychiatrist or social worker—either at the time of her initial surgery or later. This woman was visited in the hospital by a psychiatrist only when she became so completely hysterical that she was threatening to jump out the window.

It seemed extraordinary that these women had never had any opportunity to talk about their problems of self-image and their sense of deprivation with some kind of trained professional in the mental health field. I couldn't believe the mental health people were ignoring this area of emotional distress. In fact, I knew that the video tape I had made for the Department of Psychiatry at Beth Israel Hospital was being used as a teaching film. But that was the only clue I had to any link between psychiatric support and the mastectomy patient, and it was a pretty tenuous link.

What about counseling sessions, rap groups, group therapy to help women face the loss of a breast? Did such things exist? I had learned about the depression and mourning following mastectomy but I had seen no documentation by the professionals in the field or in case histories.

It seemed as if women were still being left to sink or swim emotionally, as I had been, at this terrible crisis in their lives. But had the seven years since my mastectomy been put to good use and a network of supportive services begun to get established?

To find out, I went back to the medical library and the interview circuit, and I learned first that what's been written about the psychology of breast loss is extremely skimpy, considering the extent of the problem. Articles on the emotional aspects of mastectomy, from what I could see, have averaged no more than three or four a year over the last twenty-five years in the publications read by physicians—not three or four in each publication, but in all the medical journals put together —and maybe one a year, if that many, in those read by nurses.

The second thing I learned is that the availability of psychological services to the patient varies enormously. Some hospitals, particularly on the West Coast, have extensive programs that include counseling by a psychiatrist or psychiatric social worker and group therapy sessions led by highly trained professionals. In these programs, women and sometimes their families, too, are encouraged to explore their feelings, express their anger and anticipate the emotional ups and downs that are likely to follow their operation.

In most hospitals, however, the only counseling is that offered by the Reach to Recovery volunteer, a woman who has already undergone mastectomy herself. The very presence of the cheerful, outgoing volunteer provides a measure of therapy. Her explanation of exercises to promote physical rehabilitation and her display of various prosthetic forms to go inside the bra are also morale builders.

The chief thrust of Reach to Recovery, the brilliant inspiration of its founder, Terese Lasser, is to remind the mastectomy patient that she is not alone. This is an indispensable service, and for many women it is a turning point in their recovery. But for others it may not be enough. And those needing deeper or more professional counseling seem to be rarely served.

The third thing I learned is that even though the medical literature is limited and therapy scarce, the link between breast loss and emotional disturbance is fully and thoroughly documented.

As far back as 1952 a lengthy article in the *Journal of the American Medical Association* explored the psychological problems of adjustment to cancer of the breast. The authors, who had studied fifty mastectomy patients at the Chicago Tumor Institute, pointed out that a woman's breasts are among her prized possessions and have two major psychological meanings. As the outward evidence of her femaleness and as symbols of glamour and attraction, they have sexual significance. As milk-bearing organs, they have symbolic connection to motherhood.

The authors state, "The breast, therefore, is the emotional symbol of the woman's pride in her sexuality and in her motherliness. To threaten the breast is to shake the very core of her feminine orientation."

That kind of statement always strikes me as being similar to a sociologist's discovery, after extensive research, that poverty is related to lack of money. Of course a woman is shaken to the core when her breast is threatened. Every woman alive knows that. But it is nice to hear it confirmed by properly credentialed professionals.

That same year Dr. Morton Bard catalogued the sequence of emotional reactions in radical mastectomy patients and published his findings in *Public Health Reports*. He traced the spiral of misery from fear of discovery, anxiety about treatment, panic at the time of hospital admission and fear of recurrence to nightmares, inability to eat, sleep disturbances, excessive perspiration and galloping heartbeat during convalescence.

That was 1952, mind you. One would think the word would have gotten around a little more between then and now, so that thousands of women wouldn't have had to believe they were freaks when they were overcome with distress at the thought or the reality of breast loss.

Dr. Bard and his associate Dr. Arthur Sutherland went even further a few years later and after interviewing twenty women before and after their operations, tried to fit their reactions into some kind of pattern. They found that emotional responses tend to fall into three phases.

In the first or anticipatory phase, the woman assesses her potential breast loss in the light of her childhood experiences of sexuality, her relationship with her mother during puberty and the value she assigns to her breasts. At this stage some women may experience such disruptive fear that they deny the problem and fail to get medical help. Others, who are better able to cope with the threat and seek medical attention, often feel trapped by the lack of alternatives and are numb, shocked, terrified, panicky or stunned when they hear the diagnosis.

Once she is in the second, or operative, phase the woman must confront several deeply frightening issues: surviving the surgery, dying of the disease, worrying about the effects of her death on loved ones, dealing with the loss of self-worth associated with the mastectomy. The last is a particularly strong concern for the woman who sets great store by her physical attractiveness. Many women see the loss of a breast as a threat to sexual relationships. And almost as many, according to the authors, are concerned about the prospect of never again having sexual feelings of their own after a breast is removed—a fear, by the way, that is completely unfounded.

In the third, or postoperative, phase the woman may feel lucky to be alive and at the same time show both dependence and resentment toward the health personnel taking care of her. She may feel unready to face people after her discharge from the hospital and is likely, in convalescence, to feel depression, vulnerability and fear of the consequences if she should be seen undressed.

How true, I said to myself as I read those words. And I couldn't help thinking of the woman I'd spoken to who'd confessed that she kept her bra on even in the shower—she felt that much horror at confronting her own body.

A common theme in many of the articles I read was the dual nature of the threat to a woman: the disease itself and the disfiguring surgery. Often amputation was found to outweigh the disease in the degree of horror evoked.

I'd found this was so for myself and for nearly all the women I've talked to. While cancer is recognized as a potential killer, the threat of death is abstract and vague, while the mutilation is ever present and must be dealt with daily in terms of dressing, bathing, sex and diminished self-image.

In the 1971 issue of *Cancer*, the publication of the American Cancer Society, two surgeons summed up the emotional toll of mastectomy: first, the anxiety connected with any major surgery; second and more important, the fears associated with breast loss and concern over sexual desirability as it affects interpersonal, sexual and marital relations; third, the fear of death.

The same old bitterness began to rise in me again. There it was, all spelled out back in 1971. Yet not one of the hundreds of women I've talked to all these years later had ever been told that her anxieties were perfectly normal or had been helped to work out her fears and use them constructively.

Take the whole question of mourning: research on mourning has increased in recent years, and the grieving process has been recognized as a series of stages that must be passed through before recovery can be completed. Loss of a breast is now recognized as a proper occasion for mourning. Shouldn't her doctor, or someone else, explain this to every mastectomy patient instead of telling her to stop crying, she hasn't lost a leg?

Our common sense tells us that such explanations are important, and so does a medical textbook, *Loss and Grief: Psychological Management in Medical Practice*, which points out that the response to the loss of a breast is even comparable to the loss of a person significant in the patient's life. The authors believe the patient should be able to discuss her anticipated loss and share her wishes and fears about her breast before surgery. If she is hesitant about expressing her resentment, she should be *encouraged* to put her feelings into words. And her husband should be included in this psychological preparation so his own fears can be explored along with his wife's.

One widely experienced reaction to mastectomy is the "phantom breast." The woman feels that the missing breast is still there or that she feels pain in it. In one study of 203 women, one-third experienced this sensation, which is probably caused by psychological factors but may be related to nerve stimuli in the breast area. One fascinating sidelight emerged in the study: for women who had not had mastectomies, the value assigned to the breasts decreased with age. But for women who had lost a breast, the opposite occurred.

One investigator has reported that some women are so traumatized by the loss of a breast that the remaining breast becomes a nonfunctioning organ. They refuse to let it be seen or touched during sexual activity. Sometimes their doctors will not allow them to use it for breast-feeding. And they may regard it with suspicion and dread because of fear of recurrent cancer. As a result, they are beset by a disquieting mixture of positive and negative feelings toward the one breast they have left. And they have to cope with that conflict along with everything else.

In addition to the adverse psychological effects on the woman herself, there is the impact on her sexual partner (unfailingly referred to as "her husband" in the medical writings.) Dr. Roberta Klein, a psychiatrist, explains that when mastectomy gives a woman a distorted self-view as a person unworthy of love and affection, she transmits this malaise to her husband.

At the same time, the husband may have his own fears and his own sense of frustration in trying to understand what his wife is going through and what new needs she will have for him to fulfill. Many husbands express their conflicting emotions and concerns by retreating from the situation. The wife may then interpret his behavior as rejection—especially since she anticipates being rejected. And so misperceptions on both their parts can lead to hurts, sorrows and even marital breakdown.

Early in 1977 three researchers in the psychiatry department at the University of California at Los Angeles reported on a pilot study of what mastectomy does to marriages. The investigators questioned forty-one women who had undergone surgery within the last two years. Sixty percent of the women rated their emotional adjustment to their operation as excellent or very good; another 23 percent, as good. Over half of the husbands found the adjustment excellent; one-third, good or very good.

But when the questions became more specific, the responses were less rosy. One-quarter of the women reported suicidal feelings after their operation; 36 percent had more than doubled their intake of tranquilizers since surgery; 15 percent were drinking significantly more; and others reported sleeping problems. Fifteen percent sought professional help for emotional difficulties.

Husbands had problems, too. Forty percent had trouble sleeping, 27 percent had loss of appetite and 43 percent thought their work suffered. Sexual satisfaction for the men declined; 23 percent of the women said orgasm had become difficult or impossible; and 20 percent of the men had not seen their wives unclothed since the operation. Women said that their husbands' reactions on seeing them naked ranged from "very reassuring" to "repulsed."

Women under forty-five seemed to suffer more from severe depression than those over forty-five. Couples with good relations before the operation seemed to make the best adjustments after it was done. But it isn't easy. Dr. David Wellisch, one of the authors of the study, commented, "A well-meaning husband tells the wife who has lost a breast, 'It doesn't matter, honey,' and deprives her of letting her anger out. She withdraws and acts out her feelings by twisting him into knots." Wellisch believes couples should talk frankly together, either by themselves or with the help of a counselor.

The researchers concluded that for the women, "emotional suffering appears to far outweigh the physical pain." Any woman who has been there will nod sadly in agreement.

Of course, not all women suffer equally. Dr. Max Needleman, chief of the Liaison Unit of the Department of Psychiatry at Beth Israel Hospital, the psychiatrist for whom I did the video tape, recently told a symposium on breast diseases: "The type of reaction or intensity will be influenced by the personality and character traits of the woman. We can anticipate that women whose appearance and self-image are most important to them may react intensely and violently to this disfigurement and change in body image. These are the women who are most likely to feel mutilated or repulsive, and who develop strong inhibitions about looking at or being looked at in that area."

Dr. Needleman goes on to say that women who have preexisting emotional or mental disturbances may react to this additional stress with acute exacerbations of their illness and with further decompensation. All in all, the psychological trauma can be very severe, with the occasional development of serious neurotic and even psychotic behavior.

H. C. Harrell, a nurse who underwent mastectomy a few years ago, described movingly in the *American Journal of Nursing* the violence of her reaction. She said at one point, "The threat of death hung over me day and night, but I believe that the mutilation was more traumatic. Living became so arduous I found myself preparing to die on all levels."

And she concluded with this cry from the heart: "To save a woman by surgical intervention and deny her emotional support necessary to form a different life style and accept an altered body image is a contradiction in terms."

Read that last quotation again, because it really goes to the essence of the matter. What good does it do to save a woman's life and then condemn her to a life she hardly finds worth living?

Now that the emotional suffering of mastectomy is officially recognized, what can be done about it?

14

What Can Be Done—on the Psychological Level

Any way you look at it, mastectomy is a nightmare. But there's no reason on earth why the inescapable physical loss should be accompanied by so much emotional trauma, especially when a large part of that trauma is avoidable.

Counseling to prepare the patient for what she's about to undergo and to encourage her to bring her own fears and her husband's, too, out into the open should be a routine procedure. As I've already said, I find it shocking that hardly any of the several hundred women I've talked to in the past two years about mastectomy and reconstruction received even the simplest kind of guidance in overcoming the psychological crisis of mastectomy. These women were in good hospitals, often teaching hospitals, and yet they were left entirely on their own without supportive psychological care.

Some experts have outlined such a program. In a recent issue of the *Journal of Obstetric, Gynecologic and Neonatal Nursing*, Nancy Fugate Woods, an assistant professor at the Duke University School of Nursing, reviewed some of the programs already available to help women resolve their tension and anxiety. She mentioned group sessions for patients and their families, groups for couples coping with the aftermath of mastectomy, preadmission education plans for women having a biopsy, preoperative teaching plans, rehabilitation efforts to restore physical function and promote psychologic adjustment, and follow-up questionnaires at one week and three months after discharge.

Mrs. Woods says of the objective of all such programs: "First is helping the woman express her feelings. Using knowledge to dissipate myths, avoiding false reassurance, and helping the woman anticipate the future, e.g., the normal course of grief, are important.

"Other approaches include helping the family gain an understanding of the woman's feelings while supporting the expression of their feelings and helping the woman decide what to tell the significant others in her life."

The prototype of such groups is the one at Memorial Sloan-Kettering Cancer Center in New York, called the Post-Mastectomy Rehabilitation Group. Patients begin attending this group on their second postoperative day and continue until their discharge. The hour-and-a-half sessions are led by an interdisciplinary team consisting of a nurse, a physical therapist, a social worker, and a specially trained Reach to Recovery volunteer. There are usually eight to ten patients in attendance. Some of the time is spent in exercise, some in discussion of the physical management of the postmastectomy period and some in examining emotional reactions.

Sona Posner, the social worker in charge of these groups, says, "The group format provides patients with tremendous support. They begin to lose their sense of isolation; they share a common experience, they become less alienated. Often they feel ashamed of their reactions, weak, vain, petty, as if they're not acting like strong adults or living up to expectations. Their guilt about this is often diminished when they find, to their surprise and amazement, that these feelings are shared by others. They find that their feelings of abnormality related to their body image are also normal."

When I hear a sensitive woman like Mrs. Posner speak in this way I could almost cry in my sadness for the thousands and thousands of mastectomy patients who have not received and are still not getting this kind of basic psychological support.

What a difference it must make in a woman's life to talk her heart out at this terrible time of strain and to learn from other women in the same situation and from an experienced leader that she is not alone in her grief, that nearly everyone in her situation has the same fears and angers and that distress is a perfectly normal reaction.

I think back over my own sense of aloneness at the time of surgery. The tragic stories of aloneness and alienation told me by so many women echo and re-echo in my mind. Then I begin to get angry all over again that these simple, therapeutic sessions aren't available right now everywhere. I wish someone would start to hurry—a little deliberate speed would help.

Dr. Jimmie Holland, chief of psychiatric services at Memorial, tells me that the National Cancer Institute is launching a large-scale study of the stresses exerted on the woman and her family by breast cancer, a study that will involve a thousand women at half a dozen major medical centers over an eighteen-month period.

"Once we've evaluated the stresses," explains Dr. Holland, a thoughtful, competent woman and the mother of five children, two of them in college, "then we can look into what intervention is the most appropriate." I am delighted that such a study is being undertaken, impatient for it to be completed.

Memorial Hospital already seems to have a pretty good notion of what intervention is appropriate, for in addition to patient group discussions while in the hospital, there are also evening sessions for patients, their husbands or boyfriends. Also, there is a group meeting six weeks after hospitalization for ongoing discussions with patients.

"For some couples," says Mrs. Posner, "this is the first time they've really talked about fear of death, about how to tell the kids, about sex. The group gives the man, as well as the woman, permission to be frightened, even overwhelmed. Once they start to talk to each other, most of the couples find it's not so hard to work out their problems. Some of them work out other problems, too, and a few realize they have real difficulties and need professional help. One woman asked me recently, 'How do couples ever get through a mastectomy without these sessions?' "

Quite a number of hospitals in the West have discussion groups for mastectomy patients, as do various community organizations around the country, such as Y's and mental health centers.

All hospitals have psychologists, social workers and nurses who have insight and sensitivity. They could easily be used in a supportive program that would vastly reduce the agony of mastectomy patients.

If you are in this situation and there is a group nearby, go. I deeply believe you will be helped enormously. Reconstruction is one of the subjects that usually comes out at these sessions, and sometimes a woman who has undergone reconstruction is asked to join the discussion and contribute her thoughts.

Another avenue of help is through the surgeon, whose role is central to helping a woman accept her mastectomy. As Dr. Roberta Klein has pointed out, ". . . he has the greatest opportunity to help and is perceived as knowledgeable, skilled and godlike by both the patient and the family. The patient is eager to believe in his power to cure both the body and the psyche."

Michael J. Asken, a psychologist at West Virginia University, published in the *American Journal of Psychiatry* in 1975 a review of medical literature on the psycho-emotional aspects of mastectomy. In assessing the role of the surgeon, he said, "The surgeon can engage in simple behaviors that will aid in postoperative adjustment. Psychological intervention can begin at the precise moment that the necessity for mastectomy is determined and may be effected by stressing any positive aspects of the situation and being aware of female and familial concerns and fears. The surgeon may see to it that appropriate ameliorative measures are instituted or administrated postoperatively."

To which all women can only say "Amen." Dr. Clinton V. Ervin, Jr., a surgeon in San Mateo, California, interviewed in depth a dozen of his mastectomy patients on whom he'd operated in the ten preceding years. "The mastectomy experience is a devastating one in which the emotional suffering far outweighs the physical," Dr. Ervin wrote. He wanted to know from the patients themselves more about that emotional suffering. What he learned caused him to adopt a new approach to patients with breast cancer. He decided on scrupulous honesty with patients while still preserving hope, open acknowledgment of their anxiety and depression, early discussion of the deformity that would result from surgery, concentration on the future rather than on the past and involvement of the husband at each step of the way.

Dr. Ervin followed the procedure of inviting a patient's husband to his office a day or two after surgery and discussing with him his own fears as well as his wife's concern over possible loss of love and the threat of the operation to her femininity.

"I insist that the husband hold her hand," Dr. Ervin stated in his report of his new procedure, "and tell her that he loves her, that she is the same woman inside and that a change in contour is not going to matter." Dr. Ervin also required the husband to change dressings as part of his involvement.

Some of Dr. Ervin's brand of kindness and understanding would help patients everywhere recover more quickly and more completely.

There's another step toward psychological recovery, a somewhat controversial one, that comes from Dr. Needleman, and I find it particularly interesting because in an odd way I stumbled upon it myself.

Dr. Needleman believes there should be a delay of a few days between biopsy and mastectomy. He feels that it is psychologically unsound for a woman to enter the operating room and be put under anesthesia without knowing definitely whether she has cancer or whether her breast will be removed. He says, "Under these circumstances, the patient is unable to prepare herself psychologically, with adequate defenses, for this most traumatic event."

He feels that a delay of two to three days gives the patient time to prepare her defenses and to enter the operating room for the second time with full knowledge of what is going to happen. Women who are not prepared and who awaken minus a breast are more likely, in his view, to develop feelings of distrust, suspicion, anger and rage and even irrational thoughts of having lost a breast unnecessarily.

To those who object that a delay allows too much time for worry, Dr. Needleman points out that worry is a useful and necessary method of preparing psychological defenses. Patients who have elective surgery, with plenty of time for worry, generally do better psychologically than emergency surgery patients. The interval, he feels, could be well used for support and counseling by family members, the surgeon, a case worker or a psychiatrist.

I am gratified by Dr. Needleman's favorable view of delay between biopsy and mastectomy because, as you remember, I insisted on such a waiting period for myself long before it was known to have psychological benefits. Even though the waiting days were filled with misery, I've never regretted my decision. And now I know I was working on behalf of my own mental health and not just stubbornly battling a hospital routine.

Finally, we come to another suggestion of Dr. Needleman's for avoiding the negative aftermath of mastectomy. He strongly favors reconstruction.

Psychologically, he believes, reconstruction solves two problems: "First, it restores body image, with a return of feelings of normalcy and completeness. It frequently restores sexual confidence and makes unnecessary the inhibition about being looked at. The breast area is no longer 'off limits' and nudity no longer avoided.

"Second, and even more important, reconstruction helps end the preoccupation with ideas of cancer, recurrence and death. In some women the visible disfigurement serves as a constant reminder of the cancer and may make it impossible to give up morbid and obsessional preoccupation with cancer, cause withdrawal from relationships, need for alcohol and, occasionally, suicide."

For these reasons, Dr. Needleman suggests that reconstruction surgery be offered and recommended to more women than it is at present and as early as possible. He even goes on to say, "Surgical techniques should be modified where possible so that replacement of the breast could be available to a larger proportion of women, since there is every indication that it is most helpful psychologically and can improve the quality of such women's lives."

Back when I was searching for someone to rebuild my lost breast, I tried in many ways to put my longing into words. Now I think Dr. Needleman has done it appropriately for the many hundreds of thousands of us who have felt maimed by mastectomy.

15

Time for Reconstruction

I think the case for reconstruction has been made beyond contradiction. And while we are still in the mastectomy era, I want all women to know about reconstruction, to ask for it, to plan for it and to go through with it if it meets their physical and emotional needs.

Do I think breast reconstruction is for everyone?

No, of course not. Some women adjust beautifully to their new body image after mastectomy and proceed exactly as before with the business of living. Some cannot bring themselves to face the strain of additional surgery, no matter how appealing the goal of a restored body. Some are so happy to be alive after their ordeal with cancer that nothing else seems important. And some, with strong religious convictions, accept their loss of a breast as part of God's plan for their lives.

No one is suggesting that any of these women force herself or be forced into the operating room to have the lost breast put back.

In addition, there is one particular group of women, eager for reconstruction, who probably ought to be discouraged. These are the unhappy women who look to a face-lift, nose straightening, breast augmentation or reconstruction or other form of plastic surgery as a means of curing deep-seated personality problems. Plastic surgeons try to be on the alert for patients motivated by fantasies or unreal expectations and will usually either decline to operate or suggest counseling or psychotherapy before a final decision is made.

But for the many thousands of women who feel deprived and devalued as a person and as a woman by the mastectomies they have undergone, and for the thousands more who will face this sense of loss in the years immediately ahead, I believe reconstruction can restore the longed-for sense of wholeness.

To make reconstruction as universally available as I believe it should be, certain steps must be taken. These steps involve breast surgeons, plastic surgeons, hospital administrators, manufacturers of prostheses, medical insurance officials and the patients themselves.

Surgeons, whether they are general surgeons or breast specialists, should alert their mastectomy patients to the possibility of reconstruction.

Dr. Millard, as a plastic surgeon, has pointed out to breast surgeons that there is an extra dividend for them if they accept the principle of reconstruction. He told a meeting of surgeons in Toronto in 1975 that the cancer surgeon "is the *hero* of the cure but ever the *villain* of the mutilation. Once he explains to the patient that she need not go through life mutilated— or, as these patients often express their condition, as 'half a woman'—he brings her hope. Many women may never bother, but at least they know their surgeon feels it can be done and, in so saying, he implies faith in their cure."

Dr. Cronin, the plastic surgeon who devised the silicone implant, suggested in a recent issue of the *Journal of Plastic and Reconstructive Surgery* several steps the breast surgeon can take to make reconstruction more feasible. Whenever the surgeon can possibly do so without compromising the basic excision of the cancer, Dr. Cronin believes he should preserve the pectoral muscle, use a transverse incision, bank the nipple, avoid excessive skin excision and do meticulous closure.

The closure—the final sewing up of the wound after the breast has been removed—is important. A careless or hasty closure will often result in a rough, heavy scar; a more careful closure will leave a neater, less prominent scar. Since this scar, even after it has faded with time, remains forever visible on the reconstructed breast—the breast implant is inserted beneath the old mastectomy scar—the patient wants minimal scarring.

It is not unknown in medical annals—in fact I suspect it is quite common—for the breast surgeon to step aside when the major and most critical part of the operation is completed and to let a less experienced assistant sew up the wound. As a result, many women end up with jagged gashes instead of hairline scars across their chests.

In some cases women armed with advance knowledge of reconstruction now ask to have their plastic surgeon close up the mastectomy wound. In other instances, cancer surgeons are vying with plastic surgeons to produce closures that are models of neatness and precision.

However it is accomplished, a woman is entitled to the absolute minimum of scarring. If the breast surgeon and plastic surgeon work together, so much the better. The key to successful reconstruction is a team approach by breast and plastic surgeons.

To some breast surgeons, particularly leading ones who have been stars in their own right, the idea of working in tandem with someone else does not fill them with enthusiasm. But surgeons and anesthesiologists have traditionally worked as a team. And there has always been a high degree of cooperation between surgeons and pathologists. Now, it is the turn of the plastic surgeon.

Dr. Kenneth A. Marshall, a plastic surgeon in Boston, spoke up in favor of the team approach in an editorial early in 1977 in the *Journal of Surgery, Gynecology and Obstetrics*. He wrote, "Now is the time for surgeons doing operations for cancer and those doing reconstructive plastic procedures to confront all of these problems as a cohesive team. Those most experienced in each of these fields must convene, discuss and agree on criteria and protocol for the timing of these procedures . . . While the surgical extirpation of cancer must take priority, more consideration must be given by surgeons performing operations for cancer and by those performing reconstructive procedures to an over-all plan and goal of management."

Dr. Marshall concluded: "In this era of informed consent with public clamor for more and better care and government scrutiny of all medical activities, we, as a profession, have been prodded into rethinking many surgical habits. Postmastectomy reconstruction of the breast needs to undergo just such a reexamination."

In Israel, as I understand it, such a reexamination has already been made, and it is common practice for the surgeon and the plastic surgeon to work together. While one cuts off, one is thinking about restoring. The patient benefits from the two different views focused on the single problem of breast management. It's a beautiful idea and should prevail in this country and wherever women undergo breast surgery.

I think hospitals can encourage this kind of teamwork through interdisciplinary conferences and through coordinators who already exist to bring together surgical teams for complex operations. For example, when a patient's face is being rebuilt as a result of a birth defect or an accident, plastic surgeon, neurosurgeon, eye surgeon, vascular surgeon and dental surgeon frequently participate in the same operation. The same spirit of cooperation should be applied to the breast cancer patient.

The next need is greater diversity and choice in silicone prostheses for breast reconstruction. As the procedure becomes more widespread, the usual rule of supply and demand will encourage suppliers to provide implants of varying sizes, shapes and densities. But as usual, I am impatient and would like to see faster progress. There is need, for example, for the development and perfection of a prosthesis that has a somewhat concave contour to its curve above the nipple. Very few women past early youth have breasts that resemble a globe or half of a sphere. Far more common is the breast that curves outward like a ball or sphere below the nipple and curves gently inward above the nipple. I don't see why it should be so difficult to reproduce this silhouette in a prosthesis. We also need more intensive research on types of prostheses shaped to fill in the disfiguring hollows left by a radical mastectomy as well as on prostheses that would better resist contracting under the pressure of internal scar formation.

Now we come to the patient. Obviously she has a right to know that reconstruction is available. If she hasn't found out about reconstruction on her own in advance, she should most certainly be told at the time of the first serious suspicion of cancer when a biopsy is ordered. Every woman is then perfectly free to accept the suggestion of reconstruction or to reject it, to ignore it or welcome it, to tuck it into the back of her mind for consideration later, to embrace it eagerly at the outset and discard it afterwards.

I don't care how a woman reacts to the thought of reconstruction or whether she acts on it or not.

I want her to know. I think this is the minimum right of every patient.

As a matter of fact, a group called Women for Women, a nonprofit organization dealing with problems associated with breast cancer which was formed on the West Coast, has issued a Breast Cancer Patient's Bill of Rights. I had intended to quote here only the right relating to reconstruction, but as I read over the dozen points that are listed I find them so pertinent and well expressed that I am going to share them all with you:

1. The right to receive a simple and clear diagnosis of her condition.

2. The right to receive all available diagnostic procedures and a complete work-up prior to surgery.

3. The right to have the consent form clearly explained to her before she signs it.

4. The right to have the biopsy performed first (under local anesthesia), including the right to see the pathologist's report and to have it explained to her. Surgery may be performed on a later date.

5. The right to be aware that for certain patients the future

option of reconstructive plastic surgery exists and to have the surgeon take that option into consideration.

6. The right to receive consideration from the surgeon and other medical personnel for the physical and emotional trauma she is undergoing.

7. The right to receive a satisfying explanation as to why the surgeon has decided on a particular surgical procedure rather than a less mutilating one.

8. The right to receive an explanation of any modes of postsurgical treatment—radiation therapy, chemotherapy, immunotherapy, etc.—that will be employed and why it was chosen.

9. The right to be referred to a therapist for physical or psychiatric therapy following surgery.

10. The right to receive competent follow-up care after surgery and to know who is going to be responsible for that care.

11. The right to be referred to a self-help group, such as Women for Women, for assistance with the personal problems that they are best equipped to help her solve.

12. The right to be always treated as an adult.

That brings us to money. The right to reconstruction is meaningless unless the patient can afford it. Reconstruction is not cheap. The surgeon's fee ranges from about $500 to perhaps ten times that for difficult and complex cases. In addition, there is the cost of hospitalization. The insert costs from $100 to $300, or up to $1,000 for a custom design.

At the time of this writing, more than half of the Blue Cross plans in the United States cover hospitalization for reconstruction.

The only way you can know whether you are covered is to check your policy or call your Blue Cross/Blue Shield office. The same goes for group health insurance plans or any other insurance coverage you may have. Check to find out.

Blue Cross/Blue Shield covers reconstruction in New York State. In Massachusetts coverage was recently withdrawn, but was reinstated when protests mounted. New Jersey recently included reconstruction in its Blue Cross/Blue Shield programs for a year and then expects to reevaluate the situation. Let's hope the decision will be to extend coverage permanently for all policy holders.

Changes can be made. In Iowa a courageous nun, Sister Mary Gervase, the administrator of Mercy Hospital in Des Moines, served on the board of Blue Cross. Though she had not had breast cancer herself, she was outraged that women had to pay for reconstruction when men were reimbursed for penile implant. She fought this sexist ruling and won—but only temporarily. Sister Mary subsequently died, and the rule was reversed.

The trend among insurers is definitely toward covering reconstructive surgery. And as the demand increases, women and their doctors will undoubtedly force the hand of laggard insurers. Dr. Kurt Wagner of Los Angeles believes doctors have a moral obligation to attempt reconstruction on any woman who asks for it, whether she has funds or not. The only course now for a woman without funds is to see if she can get the operation done in the clinic of a teaching hospital.

Several times in the last few pages I referred to sexist attitudes of doctors and hospitals. Many people have asked me if I believe that mastectomy is an act of aggression by male surgeons against female patients. I do not. I do not subscribe to this view held by some feminist extremists. I do not believe that surgeons, either consciously or unconsciously, are cutting off women's breasts to express their hostility to women. This is nonsense.

On the other hand, I do believe that there's truth in the statement that if the need to amputate a man's penis or testicle were as common as the need to cut away a woman's breast, massive research for alternative procedures would long since have been undertaken.

I do not want to undermine any woman's confidence in her doctor. Cancer is bad enough without its treatment becoming entangled in a war between the sexes.

But I do think every woman has the right to a doctor who will treat her with dignity and sensitive understanding of the great feeling of deprivation she is suffering.

And I think every woman who undergoes mastectomy should know that she has a *right* to feel deprived.

Netta Grandstaff, Ph.D., research associate with the Department of Family, Community and Preventive Medicine at Stanford Medical Center in California, recently listed the normal responses to breast cancer: denial, anger or frustration, depression, a sense of grieving or mourning, and fear.

"It should be stressed again and again," she observed, "that these are not psychopathological responses; these are natural and normal reactions to the emotional stress induced by having breast cancer and a mastectomy."

Further, I think everyone concerned should remember that reconstruction is lifesaving in that it removes the fear of permanent mutilation which causes some women to defer seeking treatment when they suspect a problem in their breast. With all the recent publicity about the side effects of mammography for women under fifty, and with the shocking revelations of unnecessary mastectomies because of inaccurate interpretation of biopsies, it is not surprising that many women are confused and uncertain about which way to turn.

Some may make the terrible mistake of delaying seeing their doctor. Or, worse still, some may refuse treatment. As Dr. James O. Stallings, a plastic surgeon of Des Moines, Iowa, puts it, "Many women would very likely be seen for earlier diagnosis and treatment if they knew there was hope of reconstruction in the future."

What I ask is that doctors and patients be aware of the possibility and benefits of breast reconstruction after mastectomy. That all necessary steps be taken to make reconstruction available and affordable to women who need it. That women who feel as deeply scarred emotionally as they are physically after the amputation of a breast know that to a certain extent what was lost can be restored to them.

It is possible to be whole again.

16

Questions Most Frequently Asked about Breast Reconstruction

Some of the questions that follow are those that women ask me. Others are questions they ask their doctors. Still others are those they would ask their doctors if they had the nerve. I've answered the questions on the basis of my own experience and from the research I've conducted among women, among surgeons and in the library. The answers are offered solely to broaden your knowledge and are not to be interpreted as medical advice.

How soon after mastectomy can I have reconstruction?
Most plastic surgeons prefer to wait from six to twelve months for complete healing and softening of tissues.

Why can't I have a reconstruction at the same time as the mastectomy?
Most surgeons find it doesn't work well. Besides, the mastectomy is often an "emergency," with minimum lapse of time from lump to biopsy to mastectomy, while the rebuilding requires planning and choices among various options. The consensus among surgeons is that reconstruction is more likely to be successful with the delay of a half year to a year.

Is it too late to reconstruct twenty years later?

It's almost never too late to reconstruct. Plastic surgeons have operated on women in their seventies, even eighties, and as long as thirty years after the original mastectomy.

Is there any danger of stirring up malignancy?

There seems to be general agreement in the medical profession that at the present time we have no evidence that such danger exists. The American Cancer Society, known for its conservative views, now approves reconstruction as an option for women who have undergone mastectomy and who are suitable candidates.

Suppose another cancer gets started in the rebuilt breast. Will the reconstruction make diagnosis difficult?

Such a recurrence is not likely, but if it happens, it can be detected in a mammogram or seen or felt by regularly checking the skin over the implant.

Will a reconstruction in any way reduce my life expectancy?

Not so far as is known. On the contrary, it might increase it by removing the anger, depression and the susceptibility to accidents and illness that often accompany despair.

I've had both breasts removed. Is reconstruction possible?

Yes, and often it is easier than rebuilding just one, since balance and symmetry are more easily achieved.

I've had radical surgery. Is reconstruction possible?

It's more difficult but possible. Make sure to see a good plastic surgeon experienced in this procedure.

I've had severe burns on my chest from radiation treatment after mastectomy. Is reconstruction possible?

Again, consult a good, experienced plastic surgeon.

My doctor says my operation was a modified radical. Is that the kind that can be reconstructed?
Yes, that's the type of surgery that lends itself well to reconstruction.

I'll be on chemotherapy for another six months. Can I have reconstruction?
Your doctor will probably want you to wait until you've completed the chemotherapy.

Will I have cleavage after reconstruction?
Not the kind you get with deep, full breasts because the reconstructed breast is limited in size. You will have about the same kind of cleavage as a medium-breasted woman.

Is the operation painful?
There's some discomfort in all surgery, but I'd say it's minimal in breast reconstruction. I did have quite a bit of discomfort the first few days after the implant was inserted, but it was quickly forgotten.

Will I have permanent scars?
You're not going to escape scarring altogether, but good plastic surgeons are almost wizards at leaving only hairline scars that fade with time. Your most prominent scar will probably be your mastectomy scar.

Why does the cancer surgeon have to leave such a prominent scar?
He doesn't always have to. In the past, when the entire emphasis was on eradicating the malignancy, nobody gave much thought to scars. But now that more women are concerned with their body image after surgery and reconstruction is more widely available, some cancer surgeons are doing neater and finer closures that leave less noticeable scars. Once in a while a patient arranges to have a plastic surgeon present

at the mastectomy to take over the final stage of closing the incision.

Can I have a baby after reconstruction?
Nothing in the reconstruction itself should stop you from having a baby. But before you make the decision to have a baby, you may want to discuss with your own physician the hormonal changes that accompany pregnancy and to have them evaluated in the light of your previous history of cancer.

Can I nurse a baby on the reconstructed breast?
No. There are no mammary glands and there will be no milk.

Will there be sensation in the breast and nipple?
Not as before, but women tell me they regain some sensation. Although the reconstructed breast remains inert, some report a slight degree of skin sensation. Others say the feeling is reflected on the chest wall. Perhaps the new breast can be sensitized mentally.

What about sensitivity in the labia if they take tissue to make a nipple?
There is usually no loss of sensitivity; only a very small amount of tissue is taken.

Will I be able to wear low-cut dresses?
I would say certainly, if you had reconstruction after a modified radical. If you had a radical and if the pectoral muscle area was reconstructed, you will be just slightly limited in what you can wear, but you may still have some hollowness under the arm and may prefer a dress that gives more coverage in that area.

Will I be able to wear a bikini?
If you had a modified radical with a horizontal incision and if your implant was inserted from below the breast, you'll be able to wear a bikini with no scarring visible at all. If, however,

your mastectomy incision was vertical or oblique, some scarring may show below the bikini bra. After a radical, only the exceptional reconstruction is sufficiently scar-free for a bikini. But if you're intent on wearing a bikini, I wouldn't be clutched up about some small scarring being visible. Lots of folks walk around with scarring of one kind or another.

My remaining breast is large and pendulous. How can the surgeon match it in reconstruction?
He can't. But he can reduce it to the size and contours of the reconstructed one.

I've always regretted that I had such small breasts. Now I'm having reconstruction. Can the other one be enlarged?
Yes, it can. But don't expect a deep, lush bosom because the surgeon will be limited by the size of the implant he can make room for on the mastectomy side.

Will my new breast have a nipple?
Not at the outset, but in a few weeks or months or at the time of the reduction of the other breast, the surgeon will make a nipple-areola for you.

Why can't the nipple be put on at the same time as the reconstruction?
It's been tried, but the nipple doesn't seem to "take" as well.

How do they make a nipple?
You should think of it as the nipple-areola, the whole pinkish circular area with the nipple in the center. It can be fashioned from tissue taken from the outer lip of the vagina or from part of the remaining nipple-areola on the other side, or your original nipple can be saved by having it banked into your groin at the time of the mastectomy and then restored to its proper position after reconstruction.

Who decides which procedure to follow?
In the case of banking your own nipple, the cancer surgeon makes the decision. For other methods, you and your plastic surgeon can discuss the options and make a choice.

My friends have read about reconstruction and are pressuring me to have it done. But I don't really feel the need. What should I do?
Do whatever *you* want. If you're happy and have made a good adjustment, fine. Stay as you are. You can always change your mind at a later date and have the reconstruction then.

My cancer surgeon is strongly opposed to breast reconstruction, but I would like to be rebuilt. What should I do?
If your surgeon's opposition is based on something specific in your health situation, you should respect his judgment or have it confirmed by another surgeon. If, however, he's opposed only because he considers the operation frivolous or unnecessary, you should try to explain to him the intensity of your need. Perhaps your last discussion with him took place some time ago and he's more favorably disposed now. If he's still unalterably opposed, you may want to get an opinion from another doctor.

My husband, my mother, my children, my friends all think I'm crazy to want reconstruction. What should I do?
It's *your* body. In my case, I went ahead in spite of opposition and indifference from my family.

My doctor says only a very neurotic woman needs a reconstruction to prove her femininity.
I disagree with him. It is *not* neurotic to want to be whole again and to recapture the body image you had before cancer surgery.

Are you satisfied with the results you got from reconstruction?
I'm more than satisfied, I'm delighted.

I'm still not clear about this—does the reconstructed breast look and feel like your natural breast?

Your reconstructed breast is unlike your natural breast in that the texture is firmer and also it usually remains inert. It does not move or flow like your natural breast. But it looks pretty good and it's certainly a fine substitute and a great improvement over having a breast missing. I might add that with time it has become almost as soft as my natural breast.

I've already had reconstruction, and now I'm trying to get up the courage to have the other breast reduced. Why am I having so much trouble making up my mind?

It's only natural because it *is* a very hard decision to make. I can only say I'm awfully glad I got up my courage and went ahead. Now I am not involved with any contrivance and I have symmetry.

Do you feel self-conscious when you show your reconstruction to other women?

Not really. Either I think of it in a medical context or else the woman and I have achieved such closeness, even though it may just be momentary, that it is the kind of sharing experience that happens without self-consciousness.

How much does reconstruction cost?

It depends on the type of reconstruction and where you have it done. A leading plastic surgeon in Boston charges $500 per breast, plus about $100 for the prosthesis. A top New York surgeon's fee averages about $1,500 for each breast. Another New York surgeon's average fee is closer to $3,000. Charges are usually in the lower range in smaller communities and outside the New York and California areas. The multiple operations following a radical mastectomy or required by radiation burns may cost considerably more.

Will my insurance pay for reconstruction?
Sometimes yes, sometimes no. In a number of states, including New York, California and Massachusetts, Blue Cross/Blue Shield covers breast reconstruction. You will have to look at your own policy and check your local Blue Cross/Blue Shield office. Prepaid health plans vary in their coverage. Check yours. Private hospitalization and disability policies also vary. Again, check yours. The trend is to extend coverage to include reconstruction.

My insurance plan doesn't cover and I can't possibly afford the high fee. What can I do?
Talk to your doctor and find out if the operation can be done in the clinic of a teaching hospital. In that event, the resident does the surgery (under the supervision of the surgeon); there is no surgical fee; you pay from $100 to $125 for the prosthesis, from $200 to $300 if it has to be custom-designed.

How long will I have to stay in the hospital?
Today, for a simple reconstruction the average stay is two to three days. The more complex ones take longer and often require multiple hospitalizations extending over a year or more.

How long does the operation take?
Usually about an hour, a little longer if there are special details or any complicating factors.

Why is general anesthesia necessary?
It is not necessary, and a few surgeons do the simpler reconstructions under local anesthesia. But general is usually preferred for the patient's comfort and to keep the patient properly immobilized.

Who is a suitable candidate for reconstruction?
Dr. Harvey A. Zarem, of the Division of Plastic Surgery of the University of California at Los Angeles School of Medicine, told a meeting of the Pacific Coast Surgical Association

recently, "When the breast has been adequately removed, when there is no evidence of any distant metastases, and when the surgeon has every reason to think that all of the tumor has been removed, there seems to be little contraindication to undertaking breast reconstruction."

Most doctors are opposed to reconstruction for women undergoing chemotherapy. One of the reasons for this caution is that chemotherapy is thought to hinder wound healing.

Is a reconstructed breast really a breast?
No, it's not. Dr. Kurt Wagner of Los Angeles describes it as a facsimile of a breast and says, "It will be an internal prosthesis. It will be a falsie on the inside, never more or less. But whatever it is, it does a woman a world of good."

Did nipple sensitivity return to your reduced natural breast?
It did to some extent. The quality of sensitivity is not really as it had been, but it's there.

Is a reconstructed breast used in love-making?
Most women report that during love-making its presence is ignored, although there is pleasant skin sensation.

Can anything be done about bad mastectomy scars?
Some plastic surgeons do restorative surgery to smooth out the scars before the reconstruction is done.

If you had to do it again, would you have reconstruction?
Yes, of course. It has changed my life and the life of every woman who has suffered from the mutilation of mastectomy.